THE FARR
DISEASE

THE FARR
DISEASE

One Family's 150-Year Battle Against ALS

DAN SWAINBANK

MARGATE
B O O K S

The Farr Disease
One Family's 150-Year Battle Against ALS

Copyright © 2015 by Dan Swainbank

ISBN 978-1-9384064-8-5

1. Medical history. 2. Vermont history. 3. ALS.
4. Amyotrophic lateral sclerosis. 5. Familial ALS.

Margate Books
A division of Brigantine Media
211 North Avenue
St. Johnsbury, VT 05819
Email: neil@brigantinemedia.com
Website: www.brigantinemedia.com

On the cover, from left to right:
Wesley Ora Farr, Frank Leslie Farr, Tennie Toussaint,
Clara Langmaid, Rena Longchamps, Kelly Ralston, Mary Prior,
Dennis Myrick, Clif Langmaid, Curtis Vance

Dedicated to the memory of:

Tennie Toussaint
Clara Langmaid
Williamina Penniman
Rena Longchamps
Kelly Ralston
Kenneth Ralston
Mary Prior
Dennis Myrick
Clif Langmaid
and
Curtis Vance

All proceeds from the sale of this book, after expenses, will go to:
ALS Research at Massachusetts General Hospital,
Boston, Massachusetts.

Contents

Introduction

In September of 1880, a forty-seven year old farmer from Sutton, Vermont named Erastus Farr somehow made his way to Montreal and the offices of Dr. William Osler at McGill University. Mr. Farr went to Montreal hopefully for treatment of symptoms of progressive muscular atrophy. Described by Osler as a "tall, large-boned man of exceptional muscular development," Erastus Farr had been a hard worker, never seriously ill, but several months before visiting Dr. Osler he had noticed twitching of the muscles in his left buttocks and thigh, and then his left leg had become progressively weaker, and as Dr. Osler observed, considerably smaller than his right leg. "In walking, the patient requires the use of a stick and drags his left leg very much," Osler later wrote in an article entitled "Heredity in Progressive Muscular Atrophy as Illustrated in the Farr Family of Vermont." In the article, Osler reported on the case of Mr. Farr and of his family.

Erastus Farr remained in the Montreal hospital for a month and received treatments of electric current. Dr. Osler noted little benefit to the patient; although the patient said he did feel better. Interviewing Erastus Farr, however, for his family history, Dr. Osler learned that Erastus was not the first of his family to be afflicted with these symptoms. In fact, thirteen individuals in two generations had been affected, nine of whom had died, including Erastus's father, an uncle and an aunt, Erastus's own brother and sister, and four cousins. In addition to himself, Erastus reported, his brother Wesley at age forty-two was showing symptoms, and two other cousins. The disease had decimated his family. Dr. Osler concluded his article:

> *Thus, of the thirteen members of the family affected, six were females and seven males, a larger proportion of the former than is common in this disease.*
>
> *With the exception of two, all of the cases occurred, or proved fatal, above the age of 46. Of the ten instances in the second generation, five are offspring of males (Erastus and Samuel), and five are offspring of females (Mrs. Streeter and Mrs. Stoddart). The disease has not yet appeared in the third generation, which promises between 40 and 50 individuals, several of whom are over 30 years of age.*

Erastus Farr, Dr. Osler's patient, died in September 1881, one year after seeing the doctor.

"This disease," as Dr. Osler referred to it, we now know to be amyotrophic lateral sclerosis or ALS, a particular form of the disease that Dr. Osler referred to as progressive muscular atrophy. For almost as long as it has been known to physicians as a separate, named affliction, Erastus Farr's family has been battling the disease and helping doctors and medical researchers understand it and hopefully someday find a cure. In the medical literature, they are known as the Farr family.

The Farrs (few of whom are now named Farr) today live all over the country. Branches have located in Utah, New Jersey, Connecticut, Virginia, and Georgia, and a number of Farrs still live in the northeast corner of Vermont. Each branch of the family seems to have its family historian and chronicler of the disease and of its devastating effects on the family. They keep family trees, perhaps with names in color of those who have died of ALS. Their own records contain members of the family who died of some form of paralysis as early as the 1700s. They work with doctors and researchers who have a particular interest in the hereditary forms of ALS. They have become knowledgeable themselves about the disease. They come up with their own theories about patterns, causes, and triggers of ALS. They have formed small charitable trusts to raise money for treatments and to find a cure. They submit themselves for testing and, when ill, for clinical trials. They participate actively in the support of victims within the family and in their regions.

This book tells the history of ALS, including the stories of prominent patients, doctors and researchers, discoveries and developments, and steps to our increasing understanding of this disease. Mostly, it is the story of one branch of the Farr family, many of whom still live in the three counties of what is called the Northeast Kingdom of Vermont. Those members of the family who have aided me in the writing of this book include the great-great-granddaughters of Wesley Ora Farr, who was the brother of the Erastus Farr who traveled to Montreal in 1880. Wesley died with symptoms of ALS in 1891. My sources in the Farr family, as Erastus Farr did, have seen parents, aunts and uncles, a sister and a brother, cousins and a son succumb to the disease in their lifetimes. They live with the knowledge that each member of the family they know and love who is in a direct line from a parent who had the disease has a fifty per cent chance of contracting the disease themselves.

They live with the fear of the disease, but also the hope of a cure. And there is a chance – because of the identification in 1993 of their particular toxic gene – that they will be part of the cure or an effective treatment that may be developed in their lifetimes. The 150-year story of amyotrophic lateral sclerosis – the early recognition of it, the study of it, and the continuous search for treatment and a cure for it – is their story.

This story of the Farr family begins in 1880 with the visit of Erastus Farr II to Dr. William Osler in Montreal. In this chart, I am calling Erastus II's generation "Generation 2." The Farr family descendants who are the focus of this book all descended from Wesley Ora Farr, who was Erastus's brother. Farr family members who were diagnosed with ALS—or who may have been afflicted with the disease—are identified by **bold** print. Obligate carriers, those who did not show symptoms of ALS but whose children did, are identified by ***bold italic*** print. Dates, when known, are provided for those who died of ALS.

Generation

1   **Samuel Farr** (d.1865), Roswell, Russell, **Erastus** (1795-1835), Martha, **Hannah** (d. 1851), Esther

2   Children of **Samuel Farr** and Thirza Davis:
- **Erastus** (1847-1881) [Osler's patient]
- **Wesley Ora** (1838-1891)
- **Ellen** (d. 1877)
- **Samuel** (d. 1879)

3   Children of **Wesley Ora Farr** and Phebe West:
- ***Mary Matilda***
- **Frank Leslie** (1872-1932)
- Myrtle

4   Children of ***Mary Matilda Farr Gaskill*** and Tyler Gaskill:
- **Tennie** (1894-1973)
- Marjoria
- Laura
- Doris

5   Children of **Tennie Gaskill McGill (Toussaint)** and Robert McGill:

- *Viola*
- **Williamina** (1917-1966)
- **Rena** (1918-1988)
- **Clara** (1922-1962)
- Tyler
- Robert
- *Calista*

6 Children of *Viola McGill Ralston* and Errol Ralston:
- Janet
- Keith
- **Kenneth** (1942-2001)
- **Kelton** (1945-1988)
- Brenda

Children of **Clara McGill Langmaid** and Forrest Langmaid:
- *Linda*
- **Mary** (1946-2010)
- Susan
- **Clif** (1954-2014)
- Jane

Children of *Calista McGill Myrick* and Charles Myrick:
- Steve
- **Dennis** (1958-2012)
- John
- Andrew
- Cindy

7 Children of *Linda Langmaid Vance* and Roy Vance:
- Chris
- Craig
- Charles
- **Curtis** (1973-1999)
- Cary
- Carl

PART I

History
(1850–1938)

What is ALS?

Amyotrophic lateral sclerosis (ALS) is known in the United States as Lou Gehrig's disease, after the Yankee slugger and "Iron Horse" whose diagnosis in 1939 first brought ALS to the attention of the American public. In some parts of the world it is known as Charcot's disease after the French physician Jean-Martin Charcot, who named it in 1870 after recognizing the separate clinical and pathologic characteristics of the disease. In the United Kingdom, it is known as motor neurone disease.

ALS is one in a family of diseases known as the motor neuron diseases. In each variation, the motor neurons of the brain and of the spinal cord become diseased and dysfunctional. They in turn control the signals to the muscles so that over time the muscles become weak and atrophied. The term amyotrophic lateral sclerosis, then, can be broken down into its parts: *a* refers to a negative impact, *myo* refers to the muscles, and *trophic* to the decreased nutrition in the muscles. *Amyotrophic* describes a wasting away of the muscles. The term *lateral* is used by physicians to locate the position in the spinal cord of the nerve fibers which deteriorate in this disease – on the outer edge. *Sclerosis* is actually an effect: it describes the scarring or hardening of the nerve cells in the spinal cord.

ALS affects one-to-two individuals per 100,000 worldwide. That means that in any given year in the United States there are approximately 5,600 new cases and 30,000 people living with the disease.

Ninety percent of ALS cases are sporadic; they occur in patients with no known family history of the disease and no known genetic cause. In the remaining ten per cent of the cases, however, the disease is inherited. The disease in these cases is referred to as familial ALS (FALS). It is autosomal dominant rather than sex linked; it can be inherited from either mother or father. Of the cases with genetic causes that have been identified so far, twenty percent of them have been traced to a mutation on a gene found on Chromosome 21q known as Cu/Zn superoxide dismutase or SOD1. Since 1993, SOD1 families have received the most attention in the search for cause and cure. The Farr family is an SOD1 family.

CHAPTER 1

Erastus I

When Erastus Farr visited Dr. Osler in Montreal in 1880 he told the doctor what he knew of the history of the disease in his and previous generations of the family. The first case that he reported was of his uncle and namesake Erastus Farr, whom we may call Erastus I, who died in 1835, thirty years before his brother Samuel. This was the first known case within the family. A sister named Hannah also died young of the disease, at age fifty-four, in 1851. With the knowledge we now have of autosomal dominant diseases, we can assume also that either the father of Erastus I and Samuel, also named Samuel (I), or his wife Ester Streeter, was a carrier. Samuel I died in 1809 at age fifty-four.

The particular disease of muscle wasting which Osler called "progressive muscular atrophy" had been classified by 1880 and given the name amyotrophic lateral sclerosis by which we know it today, but that label has not been used very often in the Farr family cases. In fact, a review of family death certificates before and since 1880 reveals very few uses of the term. On the death certificate of Erastus's brother Samuel, who had died the previous year, the cause of death was referred to as "palsy." Down through the years the disease has been identified by local doctors as a form of paralysis, polio, dystrophia, muscular atrophy, and peripheral neuropathy. Within one branch of the family, it was known as the "creeping palsy," but, especially for a member of the Farr family who has seen the pattern and the prevalence of the disease, they are all code words for amyotrophic lateral sclerosis.

· · · · ·

Amyotrophic lateral sclerosis was characterized and named as a separate disease by the French physician often referred to as the father of neurology, Jean-Martin Charcot. Charcot and a colleague first described the disease in a French journal in 1869, separating it from other forms of muscle wasting. This achievement ran in sequence with his work on a series of neuro-muscular diseases, including multiple sclerosis, Parkinson's disease, and Tourette syndrome, which Charcot had a hand in categorizing over a thirty-three year career at the famous and important Hopital de la Salpêtriere in Paris.

Charcot's tenure at the Salpêtriere was a fortuitous and productive coming together of a number of factors. He was the right man at the right time in the right place. He was surrounded by excellent colleagues and he built his work on respect for the work of others. Charcot was the right man due to his excellent powers of observation and his strong beliefs in the need to categorize separate diseases based on groups of symptoms, and to base diagnoses on hard clinical-anatomical facts about the nervous system. He was born at the right time because advances in neurology (and medical technology, especially the microscope) were happening all over the world. In addition, attitudes toward the mentally and neurologically ill, especially those who were destitute, were changing, and the hospital to which he was assigned was being transformed from a vast asylum of misery, mainly housing destitute and forgotten women, to a first class hospital and clinic in the heart of Paris.

Charcot and his colleagues saw the vast wards and populations of the hospital as case material needing to be sorted and understood. They set out working together to visit the wards and notice the symptoms of patients, many of whom were simply categorized by one symptom, or with labels such as "noninsane epileptics." According to his biographers, the two men spent hours traveling through ward after ward and taking notes. The insane women, referred to as alienes, they left for their colleagues in psychiatry (although later in his career Charcot took a strong interest in hysteria). The women with physical ailments they began to study thoroughly. Many of these women showed forms of what was broadly classified simply as epilepsy.

It was in the period of 1861-1862 that Charcot and colleagues began to study the constellation of ailments that included symptoms of paralysis, palsy, tremors, and muscle wasting. With the Salpêtriere's vast number of patients, Charcot was able to begin to differentiate between the various diseases involving movement, including Parkinson's disease, multiple sclerosis, tabes dorsalis, and other diseases of the motor neurons and of sclerosis. Charcot had set up the Salpêtriere's first laboratory and therefore was able to take advantage of advancements in the use of microscopes to see and record the pathology of the different diseases.

One of Charcot's teachers at the Paris School of Medicine, Jean Cruveilhier had described what we now know as amyotrophic lateral sclerosis in 1853 in an article about a circus performer named Prospere Lecomte, and had also described multiple sclerosis in his medical textbooks. Medical historians have since found descriptions of ALS in journals and books earlier, but Charcot and the medical profession were unaware of them. Medical historians today, as did Charcot's colleagues worldwide, credit Charcot with clearly once and for all time distinguishing this disease from other forms of paralysis and tremor, especially Parkinson's disease.

According to biographer Georges Guillain, Charcot in 1865 examined a woman with a spastic paralysis of all four extremities. Her disease seemed to be progressing more quickly than other forms of progressive weakness. He was looking at amyotrophic lateral sclerosis, and he quickly began to see it as a separate clinical entity. Later, in his initial lecture on the disease as part of one of his informal Tuesday talks for the Saltpêtriere staff, he noted the findings as seen in autopsies, in particular the "symmetrical sclerosis of the lateral columns" of the spinal cord.

"It is on the contrary, a distinct morbid entity which merits in many respects to be placed in a separate category analogous to the primary gray degeneration of the posterior columns (the anatomic substratum of progressive motor ataxia, from which amyotrophic lateral sclerosis can be easily distinguished clinically)," he reported in his first lecture on the topic in 1868. In his lecture he noted several other telltale signs of the disease still used today to initially separate it from other diseases:

- progressive muscular atrophy

- the progress of the disease to all four extremities

- the claw-like deformity of the hands

- the bulbar palsies affected by the loss of muscle function in the tongue

- the fact that the senses and intellect are not affected

- the grim prognosis of the patients

- and in autopsy the sclerosis affecting the posterior part of the anterolateral columns throughout the entire length of the spinal cord

Charcot was also matter-of-fact about the terminal nature of the disease in virtually all patients. "There does not exist as far as I am aware," Charcot later carefully wrote, "a single example of a case where, the group of symptoms just described having existed, recovery followed."

Guillain in his 1959 biography of Charcot referred to this early lecture as "a masterpiece," which has "remained unmodified throughout the international literature, where it is often referred to as 'Charcot's disease.' " Charcot continued to study the disease among his patients into the 1880s. According to Stanley Finger, in his history Minds Behind the Brain, Charcot last lectured on it in 1888, when he presented the case of a fifty-seven year old man. As the man, in a fairly advanced stage of the disease, was helped from the lecture hall, Charcot was said to have told him that he would soon be prescribing some ways for him to get better. After the man left, Charcot reminded his students that there really was no treatment, that he had simply wished to treat the man with compassion.

While Charcot was doing his pioneering work in Paris, a young doctor in Montreal was making a name for himself. William Osler, when visited by Erastus Farr in September of 1880, was a thirty-one year old physician eight years into what would be a long, international career. The son of an Anglican minister from Bond Head in what is now the province of Ontario, Osler had studied medicine at the Toronto School of Medicine, at McGill University in Montreal, and in Europe before returning to Canada and to McGill in 1874 as a Professor of Medicine.

When visited by Erastus Farr in 1880, Osler was interested in the heredity of disease, perhaps, biographer Harvey Cushing speculates, prompted by his reading of the studies of Francis Galton in the 1870s. Osler was not a neurologist and had not at this stage written about motor neuron diseases or forms of sclerosis. Based on his subsequent article about the Farrs, it was the mysterious heredity of this disease in one family that caught his attention. The article contains no speculation about the causes or roots of the disease.

Like Charcot, Osler believed in what he called "see sickness," the power of observation. In observing Farr, stripped, he noticed the muscle wasting, the left leg smaller than the right in measured circumference, "2.5 cent" in the calves, "7 cent" in the thighs. Osler noticed the "fibrillar twitching" in the smaller leg but also in other parts of the trunk and other extremities. He measured normal sensation in the legs, and their "electro-contractility." He observed the patient walking, and then recorded the family history. Osler treated Farr for a full month in the McGill Hospital, mainly with electricity, "galvanic and faradic currents." The treatments were "without evident benefit" to the patient, Osler wrote, "though he thought himself somewhat improved."

In his article, Osler then listed and tallied the members of the Farr family who had been afflicted with the disease of progressive muscular atrophy, as he called it, thirteen members of the family in just two generations, six females and seven males. He appended a genealogical chart showing the children of Samuel Farr [I] – Roswell, Russell, Samuel [II], Mrs. Stoddard, and Mrs. Streeter – and their many children, including the offspring of Samuel [II] – Wesley, Erastus, Edwin and Matilda. Those who had been afflicted with the disease were shown in bold. "The others escaped," Osler wrote.

William Osler went on to become Chair of Clinical Medicine at the University of Pennsylvania in Philadelphia in 1884. In 1885, he founded the Association of American Physicians, dedicated to "the advancement of scientific and practical medicine." Then he moved to Johns Hopkins Hospital in Baltimore in 1889, where he co-founded its School of Medicine, and presided for a period of sixteen years over its growth into a renowned medical center. Starting in 1892, he published editions of his classic Principles and Practices of Medicine, the standard textbook for all doctors. He remained at Hopkins until appointed to a chair at Oxford University. He was created a baronet in the Coronation Honors List in 1911 for his many contributions to medicine. He died in 1919 at the age of seventy from a stroke.

Osler's article about the Farrs was "lost to the literature of progressive muscular atrophy," according to Dr. Madelaine R. Brown in her 1951 article in the *New England Journal of Medicine*. Dr. Brown's article revisited an earlier set of nineteenth century cases of what we now know as FALS, familial amyotrophic lateral sclerosis, although she doesn't call it that.

Dr. Brown's essay, entitled "The Wetherbee Ail: The Inheritance of Progressive Muscular Atrophy as a Dominant Trait in Two New England Families," describes two families from the medical literature: the Wetherbees of Gardner, Massachusetts, and the Farrs of Vermont. In addition to the Osler article, Brown's reporting summarizes the contents of six letters found in the Osler papers at the McGill University library, and medical records at Massachusetts General Hospital (MGH), where Dr. Brown worked. The Wetherbees' family history found in the MGH records includes a pamphlet dated 1874, written by a member of the Wetherbee family. In the pamphlet, a forty year old chair maker from Gardner, himself having been diagnosed with progressive muscular atrophy, tells what he knows of the family disease, known within the family as "The Wetherbee Ail," going back to his great-grandfather. He reports about his own father, who died of the same symptoms at the age of forty-one in 1846, and records in brave detail the early symptoms and the progress of his own disease.

Of the six letters found at McGill, three were written in the 1890s to Osler – then at Johns Hopkins – by sons of his 1880 patient Erastus Farr, and three were written to Osler in 1912 by Dr. Winfred Lane of Brattleboro, Vermont. Those letters tell of two brothers, nephews of Erastus Farr, both of whom had symptoms of the disease, both starting at age thirty-six. One brother had entered Massachusetts General Hospital; the other had remained the patient of Dr. Lane. "It has been ascertained," Brown writes, "that all three brothers of the patient admitted to the Massachusetts General Hospital died of progressive muscular atrophy. One sister did not have the disease."

"There is little doubt," concludes Dr. Brown, "that members of these two families had a progressive degeneration of the anterior horn cells of the spinal cord and that bulbar palsy was the cause of death in the Vermont family. In the two families described, the type of inheritance was that of a mendelian dominant for several generations."

Dr. Madelaine Brown's work in documenting the prevalence of

familial ALS, focusing on certain New England families including the Farrs, brought the family back into prominence in the medical literature and in the search for an understanding of the genetic basis of the disease, and the search for a cure. Her work is carried on today by researchers at Massachusetts General Hospital in Boston and the University of Massachusetts Medical Center in Worcester.

The most common inheritance pattern for familial ALS (FALS) is called autosomal dominant. In that pattern a child may inherit the defective gene from either father or mother. A child born to someone who has FALS has a fifty percent chance to inherit the FALS gene mutation and conversely, a fifty percent chance to avoid inheriting the FALS gene mutation.

Later research by members of the Farr family and by researchers of familial ALS have traced the Farr Disease back through time to the marriage of Samuel Farr [I] to Esther Streeter in 1784. Those same genealogical tracings have found a possible strand of the disease in the Streeter family down through the generations, in the Underwoods in the 1700s, in the Hadley family in the early 1800s, and others. In addition, records show that Samuel I's daughter Hannah married a Hiram Streeter (with the same last name as her mother), suggesting consanguinity. Hannah and Hiram Streeter had seven children, four of whom apparently died at a relatively young age of paralysis. In fact records show that between the year of the marriage of Samuel Farr and Esther Streeter in 1784 and the time of the cases described to Dr. Osler in 1880, many Farrs had died of paralysis of some form at a relatively young age.

In her 1951 article, Dr. Brown did not publish a new family tree showing tracings of FALS in the Farr family since Dr. Osler's article in 1880; however that was her field of interest and posters of her work on the family tree, used in her lectures, have been preserved. In her 1951 article Dr. Brown added a note:

> *I am indebted to many members of the Farr family but to two in particular, Mrs. Tennie Toussaint and Mr. Clarence Farr.*

Tennie Toussaint is the grandmother of several of my sources for this book, and her story is told in Chapter IV.

The Farrs of Northern Vermont came in contact with the medical establishment in 1880, but they apparently did not consistently maintain that contact during the first half of the Twentieth Century. Some members of the family were treated at major medical centers such as Massachusetts General Hospital, and some were not. Since Dr. Brown's 1951 article, members of the family have been in communication with medical centers in New England and in Georgia, and with some of the foremost neurologists in the field. Their deaths are recorded in databases maintained by Massachusetts General Hospital in Boston, The University of Massachusetts Medical Center in Worcester, and Emory University in Atlanta.

. . . . .

The Farrs of Northern Vermont – children, grandchildren and great-grandchildren of Tennie Toussaint mentioned above – have at times been able to put the family pattern of the disease out of their minds for a decade or two. Children were raised without that fearful burden, mainly because the disease did not affect anyone near them, and it has not been part of the family upbringing to sit down with children at a certain age and have "the talk." Also several of the family's loved ones who have become ill with ALS have simply decided not to be treated in large medical centers with ALS programs. That decision has usually been based on fate or faith: they understood that there was nothing that could be done to slow the progress of the disease or to cure it, and/or they have put themselves in the hands of God.

Early Symptoms

Damage to motor neurons caused by ALS occurs in three places – the brain, the brain stem, and the spinal cord – but ALS usually begins to show itself in some sort of problem with movement. It usually is detected by muscle weakness in one muscle group, such as the lower extremities, or one side, or the upper body, or in the muscles used for speech and swallowing, the bulbar muscles. First symptoms may be a weakness in one leg, or one hand, or difficulty swallowing, just general fatigue, a "foot slap," or increased tiredness as the day goes on. A patient may feel that he isn't as fit as he thought; he or she may sweat more in exertion. Roughly forty percent of ALS patients first experience upper body weakness, forty percent weakness in some part of the lower body, and twenty percent symptoms in speaking or swallowing. For one patient, a choir member, the very first symptom that was curious and frustrating was that she couldn't hit a particular note. For another, there was difficulty holding a pencil and an odd dent in the space between his thumb and forefinger. In spring training in 1938, Lou Gehrig simply felt that he wasn't hitting the ball with any thump, and he stumbled once rounding first base.

An early sign of the disease is a loss of dexterity, the inability to do simple tasks as well as the patient thought she could. Both voluntary and reflex motions seem to be affected. The patient feels clumsy at simple fine motor tasks. The muscles become spastic, that is they tense up when used in the process of stretching out the muscle; they won't stretch. They won't contract well either, so that the muscles lose their ability to allow smooth function. They "catch," and then when passively moved, they relax.

Doctors over the years have also detected a telltale sign of upper motor neuron disturbance in the big toe, called the *Babinski sign*. The big toe extends upward and the other toes fan out in response to a firm stroke of the outer edge of the sole. In the upper body, the *Hoffman sign* or the *Trommer sign* shows in the reflexes in the finger muscles. The effects of spasticity may also begin to appear in the voice, as the highly coordinated muscles allowing speech begin to be affected. The voice may sound forced or labored and articulation more difficult.

Muscles work only by contraction, so that any movement involves a balance in the exertion of one set of muscles followed and inhibited or controlled by the countervailing set. Therefore, with progressive muscle weakening and wasting, both the initial exertion and the inhibiting contraction are faulty. A muscle group may be flaccid (not working) or over-excited. Fasciculations are subtle twitches or vibrations on the body surface over a muscle. They may be very fine or flickering, not even noticeable to the patient, but may be observed by the doctor. They are found in all ALS patients at some point and sometimes are the telltale sign. Muscle cramps are a different thing, usually a lot more noticeable. They result from hyperexcitability of motor axons, and those cramps are prolonged and painful; they distort the joint and hurt a lot.

Electrical discharges usually beginning with an intention in the brain may not travel to the muscle or may be sustained and result in a prolonged contraction, a cramp. The patient's muscles do unpredictable things.

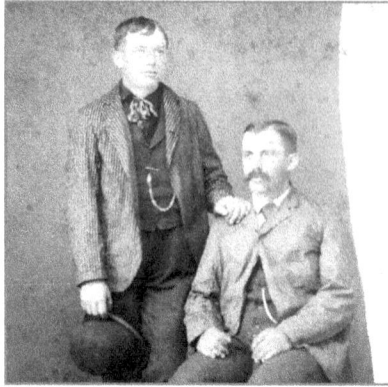

Wesley Ora Farr (seated) and his son
Frank Leslie Farr around 1889.

CHAPTER 2

Wesley Ora

When he visited Dr. Osler in 1880, Erastus Farr, then age forty-seven, reported that four of his family members were afflicted with the symptoms of progressive muscular disease at that time. They included his brother Wesley Ora Farr, age forty-two. It is from Wesley Ora Farr that my sources who still live in Vermont are descended. Wesley was one of nine children of Samuel Farr (second generation Samuel) and Thirza Davis. Family records suggest that it was Samuel II who brought the family to Vermont in 1829 from Chesterfield, New Hampshire, where he was born. His wife Thirza was born in Waterford in the northeast corner of the state.

Most of the Farrs in that era were farmers, and Wesley apparently worked in both carpentry and farming. He was living in Sutton, Vermont when he married a Sutton girl, Phoebe West, in 1870. They would have three children, Mary Matilda, Myrtle, and Frank. Birth records show that he was working as a farmer when his daughter Myrtle was born in 1882.

Growing up, Wesley probably was well aware of the family disease. His uncle Erastus (I) died of ALS in 1835, three years before Wesley was born. He lost an aunt, Hannah, in 1851; his father Samuel (II) in 1865; his aunt Eudora (or Ellen) in 1877; a cousin, Hiram, in 1878; and his two brothers, Samuel and Erastus (Osler's patient) in 1879 and 1881 respectively. By the time Wesley himself became ill with the symptoms of ALS, probably around 1890, he would have seen much and, we assume, known of his brother's visit to Montreal to meet with Dr. Osler. (The fact that Wesley Ora himself had "muscle twitching" in 1880 as reported by his brother to Dr. Osler, and yet lived another eleven years, remains a mystery.) Wesley Ora Farr died in September of 1891 at age fifty-three. His death certificate reads that he died of heart disease, but he also had symptoms of ALS and he is listed in the database of Massachusetts General Hospital as a victim of the disease.

According to Dr. Osler's account, when Wesley's brother Erastus visited him in 1880 he had reported that a cousin, a Mrs. Robinson, age forty-eight, was also affected. Her arms were no longer of any use, and she died soon after. "The disease has not yet appeared in the third generation," wrote Dr. Osler, but it soon did. Wesley's and Erastus's nephew Leon, their brother's son, died of ALS in 1906 in Brattleboro, VT. Almira Stoddard, a cousin, died in 1910. Leon's brother, Wesley's nephew, Norman Farr died in 1929 at age fifty-three.

· · · · ·

Between 1880 and 1940, as members of the extended family suffered and died from ALS in various parts of the country, the medical profession continued to learn more about neurology in general and the neurons, axons, and dendrites, which convey our intentions to our muscles. The Nobel Prize in Medicine was awarded in 1906 to two great neurologists: Camillo Golgi of Italy and Santiago Ramon Y Cajal of Spain. As described by Stanley Finger in his excellent *Minds Behind the Brain: A History of the Pioneers and Their Discoveries*, the older scientist Golgi (age sixty-three) would be justly credited with discovering, through advances in microscopic study and the use of stains, a number of features of the neurons, axons, dendrites and the nature of cells. But Golgi would have to abandon his theory of neuron growth and transmission, the nerve net theory. Honored on the same stage in Stockholm would be the man whose theories of neuron growth, directional conduction, and the structure and function of the nervous system already seemed more credible. That would be Cajal.

It was Santiago Ramon Y Cajal, experimenting with the brains of birds and mammals and not finding evidence of actual fusion of fibers at the juncture of neuron and muscle, who instead begin to believe that the axon reaches out to the dendrites of the next cell but does not fuse. The term *neuron* was introduced into the medical vocabulary in an 1891 paper by the German director of the Anatomical Institute of the University of Berlin, Wilhelm von Waldeyer. Citing the work of Cajal, he concluded that the neuron was "the anatomical and functional unit of the nervous system."

The scientist best known for his work in that era to confirm and extend our knowledge of how the whole nervous system works was Charles S. Sherrington (1857-1952). Having lived for ninety-five years, Charles Sherrington himself saw the advances in neuroscience from Charcot to Gehrig. In his long career, he coined the term *synapse* to label the functional junction between neurons, he extended our knowledge of involuntary versus deliberate muscle action, and he explained our reflexes, such as the knee jerk.

Sherrington eventually mapped virtually the whole spinal nerve system. Using monkeys, he would isolate a particular spinal root (by severing the roots on either side of it) and then stimulate it electrically, making note of the muscles that were affected. This mapping of the peripheral roots led to accurate drawings and models of the nervous system from head to toe. These drawings, once published, were valuable to doctors seeing patients with a disturbance or malfunction in a particular part of the body.

The 1910 edition of Dr. William Osler's massive *Modern*

Medicine: Its Theory and Practice provides a snapshot of the medical world's understanding of ALS in that era. First published in 1892, the multi-volume encyclopedia of all of medicine was subtitled *In Original Contributions by American and Foreign Authors.* It was continuously updated and in print until 2001. The various editions provide us with a mapping of the growth in our understanding of motor neuron diseases such as ALS.

In the 1910 edition, Chapter II on diseases of the motor tracts was written by Dr. William G. Spiller of the University of Pennsylvania. Spiller's chapter devotes eight pages to amyotrophic lateral sclerosis and includes two photographs. It provides a snapshot of the turn-of-the-century understanding of the nervous system and of the disease as understood by practicing physicians; its citations go back to Charcot and the Salpêtriere. "The French are fond of calling the disorder Charcot's disease," Spiller wrote in a nod to the great French physician. Charcot described the disease "so fully that [Charcot's Paris colleague Pierre] Marie has likened his description to the origin of Minerva fully equipped from the head of Jupiter."

Amyotrophic lateral sclerosis, Spiller wrote in 1910, is probably an abiotrophy, a disease that emerges later in life in a person who has a genetic predisposition (a form of premature aging). Spiller then described the manifestations of the disease that have been found in autopsy in parts of the nervous system, and in muscles in parts of the body.

Contrary to today's understanding, Spiller wrote, "Heredity and occupation do not seem to exert an influence," an interesting and somewhat confusing surmise since he had called ALS an abiotrophy, and because the family histories of the Farrs and the Wetherbees were part of the medical literature. Spiller mentions no work with clusters of patients, either familial, geographical or occupational.

The treatment section of Spiller's chapter is very short. "We have no means to arrest its course," he wrote of ALS. "The results are not brilliant." Strychnine may be of service, overexertion is to be avoided, and massage, passive movements, and electricity "are of doubtful value."

In Spiller's era to a large extent, if a physician had an inkling about a particular drug or other regimen (such as strychnine) he was free to just try it, especially in the case of a relatively rare and terminal illness such as ALS. In 1905, the American Medical Association had formed its own Council on Pharmacy and Chemistry. The council evaluated drugs for a fee and began to award the AMA's Seal of Approval only to those medicines it certified. Only those medicines could advertise in the association's journals. In America, the development of new treatments and the marketing of new drugs were influenced, if not actually governed, by the passage of the Pure Food and Drug Act in 1906. That act had very little teeth, but it did start a process which would eventually lead to more truth in labeling, listing of dangerous ingredients, and it provided legal definitions of "misbranded" and "adulterated." According to Suzanne White Junot, in her short history of clinical drug trials, so-called "patent medicines" (which were not actually patented) made up seventy-two percent of all drug sales at the turn of the century. The sorry state of village medicine was a triumph of advertising and hucksterism, not of science, and the patient had only his or her own skepticism as a protection against the ineffective or downright dangerous nostrums that his or her doctor (or anyone else) might casually offer.

Gradually, spurred on by successes in laboratory science, on the one hand, and by their awareness of the dangers and fraudulent claims of patent medicine on the other, however, the basic idea of clinical trials – the idea that a medicine should be proven safe and effective by testing before marketing – was growing among doctors. Progress was being made to bring the best practices of the profession into the realm of professional standards and law.

· · · · ·

In addition to reading the published medical histories and the textbooks of different eras, another way to understand amyotrophic lateral sclerosis and how it was understood and treated in certain eras is to read the biographies and autobiographies of famous people who were diagnosed with the disease. Lou Gehrig's case in 1938 first brought the disease to the attention of the American people, but before Gehrig there were other cases among prominent people. One was the renowned Jewish philosopher and theologian Franz Rosenzweig, whose biography provides a case study, not only of the progress of the disease and attempts at treatment, but also of what is now called palliative care and of the social aspects of life with the disease. Rosenzweig also was, after all, a deeply religious man and a philosopher who faced the disease with courage, faith, and sometimes startling honesty.

In November of 1921, Franz Rosenzweig inexplicably stumbled and fell several times near his home in Frankfort, Germany. He mentioned it to a physician friend, who agreed to examine him and who then told Rosenzweig that he was concerned about paralysis. As the year drew to a close, however, Rosenzweig noticed other symptoms: he had difficulty going down stairs, he had to lift his legs higher and deliberately in walking, was always in fear of falling, and he was having a hard time swallowing and pronouncing certain sibilants.

A former medical student, Rosenzweig knew that his affliction was neither trifling nor temporary. He visited a specialist, and then to confirm that diagnosis visited his friend Professor Richard Koch. Koch recorded that visit in a later memoir:

> *The diagnosis shows that even at that time the entire motor nervous system, from the cortex of the cerebrum to the muscles, was disturbed, more on the left side than on the right, that both legs were lightly paralyzed, again the left more than the right, but that the arm muscles were normal. The medulla oblongata was already affected, and thus the patient seemed doomed.*

Koch reported that his friend and patient seemed surprisingly "exhilarated," showing no signs of anxiety, instead revealing an intense interest in his diagnosis: amyotrophic lateral sclerosis. As his biographer Nahum Glatzer recorded it, "The end was expected within a year."

Franz Rosenzweig was only thirty-five years old at the time of his diagnosis. He was in a unique position to record his experiences with ALS and he did, giving a fascinating account of the physical, social, and spiritual challenges facing the patient. The story of his life, entitled *Franz Rosenzweig: His Life and Thought*, written by Glatzer, provides an account of the resourceful ways in which Rosenzweig, his doctors, and his wife coped with the disease in that era. Rosenzweig lived for eight years with the disease, a relatively slow progression, which he was able to record. Also, his upper body was last affected so that he could continue to write for a while. In addition, Rosenzweig was a realist, engaging the world as it is rather than as we wish it to be.

Rosenzweig likened his journey as an ALS patient to a train trip:

> *It's possible to "go along" just as it is possible to go as far as the railroad station, that is, up to the moment that the whistle blows and the train disappears. And one doesn't want to be accompanied to the station by just anyone. And while those who are left behind have only the grief of separation, the traveler in the window has, besides, an obscure anticipation of what waits for him. This interposes a feeling of strangeness between him and those who come to see him off.*

In the months and years to come, as his diagnosis and prognosis became clear and certain, Rosenzweig frequently referred to ALS in surprising terms, in poetic eloquence describing his reaction to his fate and his prognosis. "People think I am unhappy. They feel sorry for me. Nobody has a right to feel that. Nobody knows whether I may not be happy. I am the only one who can know that," he said to Koch.

He considered the proper sentiments for doctors, patients and visitors:

> *Doctors shouldn't take a sentimental view of death; they are the companions of the dying man, not mere bystanders. The dying themselves are not sentimental. And the bystanders are the less so the less they are mere bystanders. I don't consider myself at all a "poor invalid"; I wouldn't change places with anyone. Not with you – which doesn't mean much, since no one really exchanges his identity – but not either with my own self of a year ago. And there are few periods of my life which I would be sorrier to lose than the past ten months.*

After losing his ability to type, he relied on his wife Edith to hit the keys for him, then in the last stages to guess which letter of the alphabet he was trying to articulate. She became very good at this, and he was able to do a form of writing almost to his death. Solitary reading also became impossible, so she and other caregivers had to turn pages for him.

Beginning in August of 1923, nurses were engaged for his care. They bathed him, helped him to get dressed, turned him in bed, and exercised his limbs to help with muscle cramps. With their help, he kept up quite a work regimen: writing, reading, and thinking from about 11:00 a.m. till midnight. When in his chair, Rosenzweig's head was supported by a massive iron frame of the kind that was used in the early days of photography to hold a head still for the slow shutter. He liked to listen to recorded music during times of relaxation. This type of palliative care, designed and undertaken by Rosenzweig and his family as circumstances demanded, is all that is mentioned of his treatment. From the beginning of his diagnosis, there seems to have been the understanding that nothing could be done. Rosenzweig, as far as we know, was not involved in any experimental treatment.

Fortunately for Franz Rosenzweig, perhaps, his work was the work of the mind, his prognosis turned out to be inaccurate (he lived longer than a year), and while losing the attention of many of his friends, he gained others who accepted his situation. As he put it:

> *The radical change in my existence has driven away almost all of my former friends . . . The positive side is this: just as old friendships dissolve, so new ones are formed. The new friends are those who from the beginning have been adjusted to the current state of affairs, and who, while theoretically knowing that things were once different, lack any realistic awareness of this. They can share the new existence, as the former friends could share only the old.*

Suffering from a cold and a bronchial infection that may have been pneumonia, Rosenzweig declined rapidly in December of 1929 after eight years living with symptoms of the disease. Franz Rosenzweig died in the night of December 10, 1929 with only the night nurse at his side. His memoirs in Glatzer's collection provide a portrait of an ALS patient facing the disease with courage, perspective and dignity, coping inventively to carry on his affairs, seeing his circle of care coalesce around him, and finally saying goodbye at the station as he travels on his new journey to an unknown place.

· · · · ·

In northern Vermont that same year, Norman Farr, age fifty-three and a husband and father of two, died of ALS. The son of Samuel III, and the nephew of Wesley Ora, Norman was born in Westmore, Vermont in 1876.

In the wide world, the death of Franz Rosenzweig probably was little noticed. In the days before global mass media and celebrity – hood, and working in an arcane field, Rosenzweig would not have been a household name in America or Europe. By that year, however, Lou Gehrig was becoming a household name. Now out of the shadow of the more outgoing Babe Ruth, Gehrig was the Yankees' captain and, with his consecutive games streak, had established his public identity as the quiet but strong and durable Iron Horse.

PART II

Public and Family Awareness (1938–1973)

The Diagnosis

There is no laboratory test to provide a definitive diagnosis of ALS; rather, it is the accumulation of symptoms over time, perhaps months, which leads to the diagnosis. Usually, the weakening of muscles shows itself in one muscle group on one side of the body, such as a weak leg. Then one of the other early signs shows itself, a foot slap, or muscle twitching, or visible atrophy in one muscle group, say the right arm's biceps. A doctor, especially one who has treated a number of ALS patients, can often recognize it before the patient does.

Other possible causes of what is happening to the patient are gradually eliminated one-by-one. It is the progression of the disease itself to multiple body regions and parts of the neuron system that eventually results in the diagnosis. The World Federation of Neurology Research Group on Motor Neuron Diseases has identified four stages in the process of clinical diagnosis: 1—possible, 2—probable-laboratory-supported, 3—probable, and finally 4—definite. During this period doctor and patient wish and hope together, not wanting to make the call too soon. In fact the average time between first onset of symptoms and diagnosis is one year, largely due to the fact that those early symptoms are both subtle and painless and may have alternative causes. But eventually the call must be made. If a patient is a member of a family that has a history of the disease, of course, then the black cloud of family memory hangs over those office visits. The patient and family know, but don't want to know, what lies ahead. Even they may understandably engage in denial or hide their symptoms from loved ones.

ALS is relentless. The patient needs to be told that, but in some careful, compassionate way. As the muscles weaken and waste away gradually all over the body, the patient will be left with his or her full senses and awareness of the effects, and of the knowledge that there is no cure, and little in the way of treatment. The patient can see the future and the stages that he or she will inevitably go through leading to near total paralysis. Every week it will be something new. First he will feel out of shape, then he will develop a limp, then he will have real trouble walking and begin to use a cane, perhaps, or eventually a walker, to get around. Then one day he will find himself in a wheel chair, which at first he can propel on his own, then later has to be pushed, and so it goes. The patient at some point will be told that the average life span between early symptoms and death is twenty-seven to forty-three months. With certain genetic mutations in familial ALS patients, the prognosis is for a much shorter lifespan – less than a year. This is true of the Farrs.

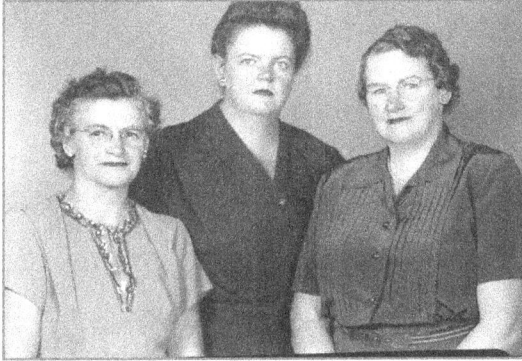

Tennie Gaskill and her sisters Marjoria and Laura.

CHAPTER 3

Wesley's Children

Wesley Ora Farr, the brother of Dr. Osler's 1880 patient and the progenitor of the Farr family line followed in this book, died at age fifty-three in 1891, probably of ALS. He lived to see the disease manifest itself in his siblings but not in his own children or in his nieces and nephews. Wesley had three children: Frank, Mary Matilda and Myrtle, who were ages nineteen, eighteen and nine when they lost their father.

Of Wesley's children, little is known of Myrtle, but Mary Matilda married Tyler Gaskill in 1892, and they had three children, all girls (hence the loss of the Farr name in that branch of the family – the branch that this book follows). Wesley's son Frank married in 1895 and he and his wife Della had three children, two boys and a girl. Frank would die of the disease in 1932, and also pass on the gene to his children. Wesley's daughter Mary Matilda lived only to the age of forty-six, dying in 1919, but did not apparently die of ALS. We know that she was an obligate carrier of the family's toxic gene, however, because one of her children probably died of ALS, and three of her grandchildren, and a great grandson. In addition, two of her granddaughters were themselves obligate carriers who lost at least one child to ALS.

What did the next generation know of Uncle Erastus's visit to Montreal in 1880? Did they read the Osler article? Probably not. In fact, after the death of Frank Farr in 1932, a thirty-year collective amnesia seems to have set in among the Vermont Farrs. There would be no deaths in the immediate family until 1962, and none in Vermont. Distant cousins elsewhere in New England and beyond may have been diagnosed with ALS, but the Vermont Farrs were apparently able to forget.

What did the Farrs know and think about Lou Gehrig when his disease was named, described, and its progress covered in the press? In 1939, Lou Gehrig became the first modern "celebrity patient" who, having established a reputation and a public persona in his or her field, then is diagnosed with a particular disease, goes public, and becomes associated with that infirmity. His many biographers, in addition to documenting his career and character, have meticulously researched the onset, course, and treatment of his disease.

· · · · ·

The 1938 baseball season was Lou Gehrig's sixteenth in the major leagues, his fourteenth as a starter at first base, and the fourteenth season of his amazing consecutive games streak as the Iron Horse. At age thirty-five, Gehrig was perhaps just over the hill from his prime years. The only category in which he had led the league in 1937 was walks, after years of leading the league in various years in home runs (three times), runs batted in (five times) and batting average (once).

A professional baseball player offers the possibility of an especially interesting study of the effects of motor neuron disease, and a first baseman handles more touches than any other fielder except for the catcher. It is all in the record: hits, extra base hits, runs, errors.

Gehrig's case is fascinating also, for several other reasons. He was the first celebrity patient, as we know them today. Played out in public, his case gives us an idea of how ALS came to be perceived (and misperceived) by the American people. He received the best medical advice and experimental treatments available during the years of his illness, 1939-1941, giving us a view of how the disease was understood in that era. Finally, because his case was relatively slow developing and described in some detail by his wife and others, and by his many biographers, we can see the stages of the disease.

He ended the 1938 season with his streak intact at 2121 games. It seems realistic to conclude, therefore, that Gehrig's definite symptoms, those that could not be attributed to anything else, began to show themselves in late summer and early fall of 1938. In any case, whenever Gehrig first began to show symptoms, there was growing concern about his baseball output late in the 1938 season, and, among friends and family out of the public eye, during the offseason of 1938-39.

Gehrig had a wonderful marriage to his wife Eleanor. They had no children and lived in Larchmont, NY. In that winter, Eleanor began to worry. Lou would stumble and trip, he mishandled small objects, and at the Playland Ice Casino, the graceful athlete looked like a beginner on skates. Eleanor began to think that he did have a neurological problem, perhaps a brain tumor.

Ironically, for such a high profile and wealthy celebrity, Gehrig did not at first get a good medical evaluation of his condition. In 1939, there were still few practicing neurologists (only ninety-eight physicians granted credentials by the American Board of Psychiatry and Neurology). According to Jonathan Eig in his excellent biography of Gehrig, *The Luckiest Man*, Gehrig first saw a general practitioner and was diagnosed with gall bladder troubles. He was prescribed a diet of raw fruits and vegetables. A practicing neurologist would more likely have noticed the telltale early signs, such as the fasciculations, that even the patient had not noticed, but Gehrig, even though he lived in one of the world's medical centers, did not see a specialist. He still planned to go to spring training, and he negotiated – without much contention – a new contract worth $35,000, a $4,000 cut. He and Eleanor headed to spring training in St. Petersburg in late February.

When spring training began for the 1939 season, Gehrig's weakness was immediately evident. Everyone noticed, including the reporters, but no one wanted to write of illness. Instead, they attributed Gehrig's futility to distraction, or to the usual spring training stiffness and lack of timing, or to age. "Rust in the old locomotive," wrote one columnist. "Father Time Scouting Gehrig," read a headline in early March. There was talk of the end of the streak, and of who would replace the Yankee legend at first base. With his teammates, he was honest. Asked by one teammate how he felt, Gehrig answered, "I can't do it anymore." To another teammate, he answered, "Like hell." On the field, he stumbled, made errors, and watched balls get by him or trickle through his legs. To the press, Gehrig admitted his failings, but attributed them to his usual poor spring training start, and to age. In spring training games, manager Joe McCarthy began to substitute Babe Dahlgren for Gehrig in the later innings.

Lou Gehrig started the 1939 season opener at first base for the Yankees in Yankee Stadium on April 20. He was playing in his 2122nd consecutive game. The opponent was the Boston Red Sox. Against Lefty Grove, Gehrig went 0-3 with two weak line drives and dropped a throw from his mitt in the act of tagging a runner. In the next seven games, he would make more errors, stumble playing first base, and fail to get around the bases to score on routine RBI hits. He looked like he was running uphill, said one writer. He ran the bases with extreme caution. In eight games, he had four hits, none for extra bases, and one RBI, and at first base and on the base paths, he was a liability. As Jonathan Eig described it, "Motions that he had once made reflexively now required slow, separate actions, as if his brain were pausing to glance at an instructional manual." His teammates tried to cover for him on the field as well as in the clubhouse when talking to reporters.

It had been understood that when Lou Gehrig, the Iron Horse

and holder of the longest consecutive game streak in baseball history, would leave the lineup, it would be his call. He was going to have to tell manager Joe McCarthy not to put him in the starting lineup, and finally on May 2, 1939 in Detroit, he did. After breakfast in the hotel, he asked to talk to McCarthy, and the two men went to McCarthy's room and Gehrig broke the news. McCarthy asked him if he was sure of the decision and Gehrig said he was. McCarthy returned to the hotel lobby, gathered together the reporters and told them. "It's a black day for me," he said, his voice choking, "and for the Yankees." Babe Dahlgren was penciled into the starting lineup, which Gehrig as captain carried to the umpires at home plate. The PA announcer informed the crowd that Gehrig's consecutive game streak was ending that day at 2130 games.

For the next forty days, Gehrig dressed and acted like a ballplayer, traveling and staying with the team. He suited up for games, talked to teammates and reporters in the clubhouse and dugout, warmed up with glove and bat, and kept up the pretense that he might return to the field, all the while knowing that he was too weak to do that. On June 12 in Kansas City, to the surprise of his teammates and manager, Gehrig offered to play in front of a particularly large crowd. Art Fletcher, filling in that day as manager while Joe McCarthy was at a celebration at the Baseball Hall of Fame in Cooperstown, NY, penciled him in at first base, batting eighth. He fielded his position at first base in the bottom of the first inning. When he came to bat in the top of the second inning, he received a standing ovation. In the at bat, he did make contact, but grounded weakly to second base. In the bottom half of that inning, however, he made two errors – dropping one throw and letting another go by him – but was not charged with an error on either. In the bottom of the third inning, he got his glove in front of a line drive hit right at him but the force of the ball knocked him on his back. When the third inning was over, Gehrig left the game and the ballpark. That evening, he said goodbye to his teammates.

When Gehrig offered to play that one last time, he had already made an appointment to go to the Mayo Clinic in Rochester,

Minnesota the next day, Wednesday June 13. Jonathan Eig speculates in his biography that perhaps Gehrig wanted to do a sort of self-evaluation just before his trip to the clinic by playing a few innings to test his strength and reactions. In any case, the game certainly confirmed his suspicions, which he had begun to share with teammates, that he was not old or rusty, but sick. He flew from Kansas City to Rochester, checked into his hotel, and walked to the Mayo Clinic.

By 1939, the Mayo Clinic had achieved the reputation that it still holds as one of the country's premier medical centers. Founded first as a family practice by Dr. William W. Mayo and his two sons, William J. and Charles, the clinic soon became a large group practice, and in 1919 was reconstituted as a non-profit organization. The clinic has grown steadily in size and reputation. By 1939, when Gehrig checked into the clinic, it had a sterling national reputation for cutting-edge care and research. The imposing seventeen-story Plummer Building with its terra cotta tower and carillon was one of the tallest buildings in the state. The clinic's staff numbered 500 doctors, including a distinguished neurology department.

Gehrig received immediate and special treatment in a hospital that was used to celebrity patients. He was seen first by Dr. Harold C. Habein. Habein was not a neurologist but he later wrote in his memoir that as soon as Gehrig took off his shirt, he could see the ravages of ALS. "There was some wasting of the muscles of his left hand as well as his right," Habein wrote, "but the most serious observation was the telltale twitchings or fibrillary tremors of numerous muscle groups. I was shocked because I knew what these signs meant – amyotrophic lateral sclerosis." Habein's mother had died of the disease just months before. Habein, not being a neurologist, however, did not tell Gehrig his suspicions nor did he consider the diagnosis definite, but he knew that Gehrig should see one of the staff neurologists, so he called Dr. Henry W. Woltman, who agreed to see Gehrig that afternoon.

Dr. Woltman was the head of the Mayo Clinic's neurology department and a nationally recognized clinician. To diagnose

ALS, Woltman had devised a checklist of symptoms, an approach still widely used today. In the manner of Jean-Martin Charcot, Woltman tended to conduct a long low-keyed interview leading to a diagnosis, and he was aware in this case that he was talking to a professional athlete who knew his body well and whose strength and reflexes were being tested every day. In the interview, according to Jonathan Eig, Woltman studied Gehrig from head to toe as he investigated which muscle groups – upper, lower, bulbar – were being affected. Then he personally tested the patient's reflexes and strength. He took out his rubber reflex hammer and tested the patient's reflexes with the knee tap. Woltman probably was convinced immediately that Lou Gehrig had ALS, but he kept Gehrig at the clinic for most of a week, conducting further tests.

Eig speculates that doctors there probably broke the news to him gradually and used the time to educate him on the disease, and to perhaps give him hope as they discussed treatment methods being tried experimentally at the time. The doctors did not level with Gehrig, perhaps planning to tell him more later. In any case, there were actually six days between Gehrig's arrival in Rochester and the official announcement of his illness.

In his book *When Illness Goes Public: Celebrity Patients and How We Look at Medicine*, Barron Lerner writes that it was during this time that Gehrig's illness was disclosed to and monitored by the public.

On his last day in Rochester, Gehrig was given a letter that became the official announcement of his diagnosis as it was disclosed to his employers, the New York Yankees, and eventually the public. It read:

> *To whom it may concern:*
>
> *This is to certify that Mr. Lou Gehrig has been under examination at the Mayo Clinic from June 13 to June 19, inclusive.*

After a careful and complete examination, it was found that he is suffering from amyotrophic lateral sclerosis. This type of illness involves the motor pathways and cells of the central nervous system and in lay terms is known as a form of chronic poliomyelitis (infantile paralysis).

The nature of this trouble makes it such that Mr. Gehrig will be unable to continue his active participation as a baseball player, in as much as it is advisable that he conserve his muscular energy. He could, however, continue in some executive capacity.

The letter was written over the signature of Dr. Harold Habein. The doctors at the Mayo Clinic did not level with the Yankees and subsequently the public. With their letter, intentionally or not, they misled the public in several ways and gave the Yankee organization some room to further mislead the public. ALS is not a form of polio, and it is a fatal disease. The doctors did accurately disclose the exact name of the disease, however, which by 1939 would be well known to the medical profession and could be explained by others. The wiggle room in Habein's letter allowed the Yankees and their fans, plus the general public, to feel hopeful, to engage in the natural shying away from terrible truths, which they did. Perhaps his doctors, to spare him the harshest of news, gave him the outside parameters. For the next two years, Gehrig's illness was public knowledge, although not accurate knowledge.

He had returned to New York and the Yankees on June 20, and soon General Manager Ed Barrow began to plan a Lou Gehrig Appreciation Day. It was set for July 4, 1939, between games of a doubleheader between the Yankees and Washington Senators. Barrow planned to celebrate the full span and achievements of Gehrig's career, and invited old teammates from the great 1927 Yankees to return for a reunion. Babe Ruth, Tony Lazzeri, Waite Hoyt, Everett Scott, Bob Shawkey, Wally Pipp and others agreed to be present to honor their teammate. Mayor Fiorello La Guardia agreed to be present and speak. They expected a large crowd.

On the day, the old Yankees crowded into the locker room and mixed with the current squad. It was a reunion with much good-natured banter. Finally Game 1 began with the ex-players in the stands. The Yankees won the first game 3-2, and the field was prepared for the ceremony. The 1939 Yankees and Senators lined up in two parallel lines streaming out from home plate. The ex-players, Mayor LaGuardia and others gathered around home plate. Gehrig emerged from the dugout on Barrow's arm and walked gingerly to home plate.

La Guardia spoke, then Postmaster General James Farley, manager Joe McCarthy, and Babe Ruth. Gifts were brought forth, including a fishing rod and tackle from his teammates, a framed parchment with the words "Don't Quit," a ring, a fruit bowl, silver candlesticks, and a silver pitcher. McCarthy gave Gehrig a heavy trophy with an eagle, which Gehrig immediately set down on the grass as if it were too heavy.

Finally, the players, dignitaries and the crowd turned to Lou to see if he wanted to make some remarks. According to Eig, Gehrig had expected to speak and had prepared some remarks, but in the emotions of the moment he was overcome and at first shook his head no. "We want Lou!" the crowd chanted, but Gehrig declined and turned toward the dugout. Then Joe McCarthy moved to Gehrig's side, put a hand on his back, and spoke to him. Gehrig then turned back toward the microphones. He held his cap in his left hand, his hands stuffed into his back pockets.

"For the past two weeks, you've been reading about a bad break," he said. His voice broke a little so that the last word came out sounding like "brag." He lowered his head and tried to collect himself. Then he said, "Today I consider myself the luckiest man on the face of the earth." He then went on to graciously compliment the fans, the Yankees organization, his teammates, others associated with the game, his wife, his parents, and his mother-in-law, to make the point that he had been fortunate. He spoke in second-person ("when you look around...") to make the point that anyone in his position would feel himself fortunate.

"So I close in saying that I might have had a bad break, but I have an awful lot to live for. Thank you," he concluded, then stepped back and dropped his head. As the adulation from the crowd poured down on him, he took out a handkerchief and wiped away his tears. Babe Ruth gave him a hug, and the cheers from the crowd continued as he trudged to the dugout and disappeared.

Gehrig kept up a steady correspondence with doctors at the Mayo Clinic, maintaining a very close relationship with Dr. Paul O'Leary. In his letters, O'Leary did not really level with Gehrig, even though Gehrig would urge him to. Gehrig's second extended visit to the Mayo Clinic began on August 20. At the end of that visit, Dr. Habein issued another optimistic report, saying that Gehrig's condition was "definitely improved."

In the fall, Gehrig started a new job. Mayor LaGuardia had offered Lou a position as a commissioner on the New York City parole board. The job required him to evaluate prisoners for release and in the process to interview them and visit prisons. He got an office and a salary and something important to do. Working for the city, he was required to reside there, and so the Gehrigs rented a home in the Riverdale section of the Bronx. It was a lovely home in a wooded area, but not a good choice for an ALS patient. Built over a huge boulder, the home had several different levels, requiring Gehrig to walk up or down twenty-five steps to get the mail, thirteen steps to get to his car in the basement garage, twelve steps to his bedroom, and three steps to get from the dining room to the living room.

Taking an active role in his own treatment, Gehrig was always seeking and receiving new treatment ideas. Fans and doctors wrote him letters suggesting remedies such as testosterone, mineral pills, or apple seed oil. Dr. Bayard T. Horton of the Mayo Clinic put Gehrig on a regimen of histamine during Gehrig's third visit to the clinic in January of 1940, "saturating his body" with the naturally occurring substance and sending him home to continue with two injections per day.

The introduction and marketing of new drugs at this time was governed by the 1938 Food, Drug and Cosmetic Act. That act was passed by Congress, at least in part prompted by the deaths of over one hundred patients who had tried a drug called sulfanilamide, one of the new sulfa drugs, marketed as a treatment for strep throat. As sold, the drug had been suspended in a solvent that resembled the chemical properties of anti-freeze and turned out to be a poison. It had never been tested on humans or animals. The new act called for the submission of safety data for the approval of the FDA before the marketing of any new drug.

The 1938 act, however, did not require researchers to show that the drug was effective, only that it was safe, and the act did not govern random trials such as those done by Gehrig's doctors, who in any case were not marketing their treatments at this stage. The act did not define and control clinical trials either.

One case that caught Gehrig's attention, as being perhaps similar to his own, was the case of a New York orchestra leader named Al Reiser. In a letter to O'Leary, Gehrig described Reiser's near recovery from what Reiser and his doctors had thought were symptoms of ALS. In writing to O'Leary, Gehrig showed his capacity for hope and his courage, but also his clear-eyed desire "to know the facts if any."

O'Leary responded encouragingly. "Al Reiser is just one of a group that have been improved," O'Leary wrote, "and there is a damn good probability that you will do likewise." In fact O'Leary even suggested to Gehrig that he ignore new symptoms that may indicate regression: as "courage and persistence in treatment invariably result in an arrest of the process such as you have." According to Jonathan Eig, Al Reiser's case was probably not ALS but a milder form of sclerosis, and O'Leary probably knew this.

In one of his letters to O'Leary, Gehrig referred to "reputed doctors," and to "these New York bastards," referring apparently to New York specialists. At that stage he was placing his trust in his doctors and friends in Rochester. Gradually however, Gehrig's case was taken over by New York doctors, one in particular. Gehrig first visited Dr. Israel Wechsler on January 27, 1940. The Chief of Neurology at Mt. Sinai Hospital, Wechsler was probably the foremost expert on ALS of his era. He literally wrote the book on neurology, publishing his *Textbook of Clinical Neurology* from 1927 – 1958. He had very strong convictions about the disease and was glad to have Gehrig under his care.

Hearing of Gehrig's regimen of histamine, and of his gall bladder treatments through diet, Wechsler became convinced that Gehrig was a good candidate for the treatment in which Wechsler had come to believe: vitamin E. Wechsler urged Gehrig to stop his histamine injections and to take five vitamin E tablets a day. Wechsler was sure that vitamins could arrest ALS and other motor neuron diseases, and in fact became convinced that it was improving Gehrig.

On March 13, *The New York Times* reported, "Remedy is Found for 'Gehrig's Disease.'"
The article reported the findings of Dr. Wechsler who had reported in the *Journal of the American Medical Association* that, as an experiment, he had treated nine ALS patients with vitamin E. Two had completely recovered, he claimed, four had shown improvement, and three had shown no benefit. *The New York Times* article also gave the disease its American name for the first time.

In May, Wechsler wrote to Dr. Woltman at the Mayo Clinic that he believed Gehrig's disease had been checked by vitamin E. By June of that year, Wechsler was reporting on the treatment at the meeting of the American Neurological Association. Of twenty patients, he claimed, nine had shown no effect, but eleven had shown improvement, two of which had completely recovered. Patient No. 4 was described as "L.G., male, age 36." That patient was Lou Gehrig. Wechsler reported that L.G. was walking better, his muscles had stopped fibrillating, his thumbs had gained power, and the disease in his case "may be regarded as definitely arrested and somewhat improved."

Wechsler's report indicates that the modern practices involved in conducting clinical trials were not in place. Needless to say,

Wechsler's formulas were not tested on animals before humans. He did not use a control group with a placebo. His and his patient's study of the results was not double blind; both doctor and patient knew what was being administered and what results were hoped for. With the attention of the world on this doctor and this patient, they got the results they had wished for and anticipated. Although the 1938 Food and Drug Act gave the FDA the authority to establish rules governing clinical trials, the FDA did not really do so until 1961.

When the 1940 baseball season began in April, Gehrig occasionally attended games, dressed in a suit and tie, and sat on the bench. In the winter of 1941, Gehrig continued to report for work downtown at the Parole Commission, but did not go out in public otherwise. At home, he was beginning to struggle with all the levels and stairs, but he liked being there, and received many guests who were often invited by Eleanor as a distraction for Lou. Many of Gehrig's oldest friends were ballplayers and reporters. He had no family circle; he had no siblings, and he had been estranged from his mother. Among his visitors were celebrities such as actor and comedian Pitzy Katz, tap dancer Bill Robinson, actress Tallulah Bankhead, and songwriter Fred Fisher. Each had been invited by Eleanor to provide entertainment and distraction. With no children, no siblings, and few true non-baseball friends, Lou Gehrig's inner care circle on a day-to-day basis was very small, consisting usually of his wife, a nurse, and his mother-in-law.

Gradually that winter, ALS began to affect Gehrig's speech and his ability to swallow. He choked occasionally on the soft food Eleanor prepared. He slurred his words and spoke very softly. Walking became more and more difficult. He walked with people at his side. Some journalists who visited him said that he was in a wheelchair; although Eleanor said that he never was.

Gehrig stubbornly continued to work long after he was really able to physically do the job. Eleanor accompanied him to his office, where she opened and read his mail for him, stamped his signature on letters, and even put a cigarette in his mouth. Finally, on April

14, 1941, she submitted a letter on Lou's behalf requesting a six-month leave of absence, still not publicly admitting the terminal disease. He and Eleanor maintained this public position even with visitors to the house that spring; although biographer Jonathan Eig suggests that that posture was taken with an ironic tone and a wink. Gehrig knew by April that he was dying; he no longer asked O'Leary about new treatments or the chances of survival.

In his last weeks, he lay completely paralyzed and unable to speak. He would often mouth the words "Fifty-fifty." On Monday, June 2, 1941, as Eleanor, his mother-in-law, and a doctor gathered around the bed, Gehrig said his last words, "My three pals," before slipping into a coma. He died at ten minutes past ten that evening.

Barron Lerner in his *Celebrity Patients and How We Look at Medicine* refers to Lou Gehrig as the first modern patient. However, the cause of understanding ALS and finding a cure for the disease was not really very well served by Gehrig, his family, or his doctors. Even the most avid newspaper readers of Gehrig's day would have been poorly educated about the disease. Gehrig's first biographer, Richard Hubler in *Lou Gehrig: Iron Horse of Baseball*, published shortly after Gehrig's death, got it wrong, continuing to refer to ALS as a form of "chronic polio."

Celebrity patients today include several with ALS and even some with FALS. They are willing to join the cause of ending their disease by allowing their symptoms to be made public. They educate themselves on the nature of their disease and the current theories and therapies for treatment or cure. They work closely with their doctors to raise awareness and money. They do not hide their ailments, appearing on television without hair after cancer treatment, or with the palsy of Parkinson's disease, or the paralysis from a stroke. As Lerner describes the process, "a celebrity, or someone fated to become a celebrity due to illness, became sick and confronted a complicated series of choices. Because of their notoriety, the patients themselves, their families, and their caregivers needed to manage not only the disease in question but how it was being spun."

There was in Gehrig's day, as there is today, a powerful force that often moves the narrative away from medical facts toward some sort of story line in which the patient *joins the war on the disease,* or *battles the disease with courage and determination*, or even *heroically conquers the disease*. To many Americans in the 1940's Lou Gehrig – his manner, his symptoms, and his best qualities – was indistinguishable from the actor Gary Cooper. Handsome, stoic and dignified, Cooper starred as Gehrig in the movie *The Pride of the Yankees*, which came out in July of 1942, the year after Gehrig's death. In the movie, Cooper asks the doctor at "Metropolitan Clinic" to "Tell it to me straight, Doc. Is it three strikes?" The doctor nods.

In the movie, then, the doctor was more honest with Gehrig than were his doctors in real life; however, in other respects the film hides from the movie-going public the grim details of the disease's progress. The movie ends with Gehrig trudging toward the locker room after his Luckiest Man speech. Gehrig would live for another two years as the disease gradually withered his strong body.

The Mayo Clinic's and Dr. Israel Wechsler's treatment of Gehrig, and the press coverage of that treatment, also established a pattern that occurs when celebrity patients are treated by celebrity doctors. The doctors and their medical centers, and the foundations and pharmaceutical firms that support their research, work closely with celebrities to raise awareness, money and hope.

· · · · ·

ALS families, and especially those with a history of the disease, while hoping and searching for a cure, are also interested in the subject of triggers. Even if they know that they are carriers of some sort of ALS gene, and that the disease is incurable, they wonder if they can avoid anything in particular that may trigger the onset of symptoms. Is there such a things as a fatal exposure, perhaps industrial, dietary, behavioral or environmental, that may bring on the fatal chain of events? In 1945, the attention was focused on the island of Guam.

Guam, one of the Mariana Islands south of Japan, was occupied by the Japanese during World War II. When it was liberated during the Marianas campaign of 1944, Navy doctors began to notice a high incidence of an ALS-like disease among the indigenous Chamorro people. Death certificates on Guam listed the cause of death as *paralytico* or *lytico*, the Spanish words that the Chamorro people had used for what looked like ALS, and records of death from the disease go back to 1815. Dr. H. M. Zimmerman reported the higher incidence of the disease in his report to the Navy Medical Officer in June of 1945.

The findings on Guam, together with other clusters in Japan and West New Guinea, have caught the attention of neuroscientists and ethnobotanists who believe that it may offer clues not only to ALS but also to Parkinson's and Alzheimer's diseases. The prevalence of ALS on Guam was fifty to one hundred times greater than in the US. The characteristics of the disease – its mean age of onset, its prevalence among men and women, all the symptoms – seemed to be identical to ALS in the western world.

Residents of Guam also exhibited a higher incidence of Parkinson's dementia complex (PDC). The local term for that affliction was *rayput* or *bodig*, which translated as slowness or laziness, testifying to the palsy of parkinsonism and the confusion of dementia. Since those earliest findings in 1945, the study of clusters and their possible causes in environmental and diet factors have constituted a promising field of study for ALS researchers. It was found, for instance, that during World War II on Guam, the Japanese confiscated food, forcing the Chamorro people to fall back on traditional, native foods for survival. They made flour for their tortillas by grinding the seeds of the cycad plant. In the 1960s British scientists, analyzing the components of the cycad seed, found that it contained a compound, beta-methylamino-l-alanine (BMAA), which was closely related to a compound that is found in Asian chickpeas and is known to cause a paralyzing disease. A plausible connection had been made, it seemed, between diet and the illness.

The mystery of whether and how neurotoxins could have

affected the brains of the Chamorro people in high doses may have been solved by an ethnobiologist from Hawaii, Paul Cox, and his colleagues. Cox learned that the Chamorro had traditionally feasted on a species of flying fox or fruit bat. The bats in turn feasted on cycad seeds, and the BMAA in cycad seeds tended to be concentrated in the bats, forming what Cox called a kind of "toxic reservoir." Testing bats which had been collected from Guam during the 1950s at the height of the epidemic of ALS, Cox found that the bats were "chock full of BMAA," according to a 2011 article in *Discover Magazine*.

How did BMAA find its way into the brains of indigenous Chamorro people in Guam? The answer, according to Cox and other researchers studying the BMAA-disease connection, focused on cyanobacteria, a very common microbe found in soil and in the roots of the cycad plant, and also in waters. It appears to the eye as the slimy green film often seen on lakes and rivers and it is ubiquitous. "Was Lou Gehrig's ALS Caused by Tap Water?" asked a headline in *The Pacific Standard* in January of 2012.

One researcher studying the effects of cyanobacteria and its possible connection to diseases such as ALS is Dr. Elijah Stommel. Stommel, of Dartmouth-Hitchcock Medical Center in Lebanon, New Hampshire, has met with some patients of the Farr family. Stommel also discovered his own local cluster of ALS patients who lived on or near Mascoma Lake in Enfield, NH. Stommel and medical students created a database of ALS patients to study any geographical patterns and whether ALS patients were more likely to live on or near water. They were. Using other Dartmouth Hitchcock databases, Stommel continues to search for clues and connections between ALS and other factors. The precise mechanism by which BMAA might make its way through the digestive process, pass through the blood-brain barrier, and get incorporated into proteins at the level at which scientists now believe that ALS deterioration begins, that mechanism is unknown. From what we know of the brain, it couldn't happen, yet something is happening. For ALS families BMAA may be more of a trigger than a cause.

"Exposure to BMAA is probably a risk factor for those who are genetically predisposed to develop ALS," says Stommel.

· · · · ·

In the 1930s and 40s in the Farr family, deaths from ALS continued, but there were not that many that registered with the northern Vermont branches. This was apparently true, even when the victim died in Vermont. One interesting case that shows the attitude within the family about ALS was that of Frank Leslie Farr, Wesley Ora's son. Frank died in April of 1932 at age sixty.

Born in Sutton, Frank had been a farmer all his life. He was listed as a farmer in 1895 when he married Della Wilson of Wheelock. At some point, he moved from Caledonia County to the Montpelier area, where he continued in farming. He and Della had four children. According to his grandson, however, due to the stigma associated with the family disease, when Frank became ill in 1931, he disappeared from view, and in fact the family was told, "He has taken off to Alaska with a mistress." A scandal of adultery and desertion was preferable as a narrative to the curse of familial ALS. His children and many of his grandchildren were unaware of the family disease until contacted by family activists years later. One granddaughter learned of the family pattern by doing basic, online genealogical tracings. She said that she grew up knowing quite a bit about her mother's relatives, but that her father's side of the family (the Farr side) was always a mystery.

Frank Leslie Farr died in Heaton Hospital in Montpelier. His death certificate lists the date of onset of the disease as April 1931; he lived one year. The principal cause of death: "Progressive muscular atrophy (Dystrophia) beginning in right arm and shoulder." Listed as a secondary cause: "Cardiac Failure Paralysis of right chest." Frank and Della had three sons and a daughter. Family activists have thus far confirmed the presence of the ALS gene in the line of one of Frank and Della's sons: Harold. Harold's granddaughter died of ALS in 2009.

At about that time, Frank's niece Tennie, Mary Matilda's daughter, age thirty-eight and herself a mother of six at the time of her uncle's death, became the family genealogist and chronicler. What she was told in 1932 is not known, but over the next few years she apparently sought to learn more and more of the patterns in the family. She would eventually realize that she was a carrier of the toxic gene. She would see much in her lifetime and is a central figure in the family narrative.

The Early Stages

ALS is a progressive disease, but both its rate of progression and the particular symptoms of the disease vary with each patient. In some patients, the disease progresses so slowly that the patient is able to continue normal activities for months or years, and may choose not to disclose his or her diagnosis for a while. Former Massachusetts Governor Paul Cellucci revealed in 2010 that he had been diagnosed with ALS four years previously, but that he was still carrying on with most of his activities. Stephen Hawking has lived with the diagnosis, and the effects, for many years, having been diagnosed at age twenty-one. Hawking turned seventy-three years old in January of 2015; he is on a ventilator today. Lou Gehrig played a year of baseball with the Yankees in 1938 after feeling the first symptoms of weakness. He then went to spring training in 1939, but he was clearly not able to play baseball at the high level that he and fans had come to expect.

The first sign of the disease, as has been noted, is a weakness in one muscle group. If the patient has the bulbar form of the disease, affecting breathing and swallowing, then a slurring of speech or difficulty swallowing may be a first sign. Some patients just feel clumsy. A patient may develop a limp which she herself doesn't even recognize at first.

There are some early signs that may indicate that a given patient has a slowly developing and slowly progressing form of the disease. A young age of onset, symptoms in the limbs rather than in speech and swallowing, and a longer period of time between first signs and diagnosis are signs that seem to correlate with the more slowly progressing form of the disease. In addition, there are factors of attitude and family support that also suggest a longer life after diagnosis, according to the American Academy of Neurology, factors such as "the presence of a marital or close supportive partner, a network of supportive friends and family, a positive attitude, a strong sense of spirituality, and a self-perception of good quality of life."

Ten percent of patients may live for ten years or longer with the disease, and maintain a good quality of life for much of their time. After diagnosis, patient and doctor may hold out that hope.

Other patients may learn through the examples of their ancestors, or based on early symptoms, that they have the fast-developing form. They may have only months left to talk and plan and develop an attitude toward their fate, and less than a year to live.

There are other forms of hope, things to grab on to as the reality of the diagnosis and likely progress of the disease become understood. Dr. Donald Mulder's approach to the diagnostic interview includes seven kinds of content. After the careful and honest description of the disease, the medical staff should try to convince the patient: that "many patients continue to lead successful lives after the diagnosis;" that "the diagnosis does not separate the patient from the rest of humanity who do not know from what they will die;" that there are medicines and devices to help him or her cope, as well as "neuroprotective" therapies, and support groups; and that there are on-going clinical trials which the patient may join. It sometimes seems as if every ALS patient has that option, which is always hopeful. Finally, Mulder wrote, "in medicine it is not possible to say never and thus there is always the possibility that the patient may improve." The patient at this moment may wish that his or her doctor either got it wrong, misdiagnosing ALS, or is a god-like healer and will bring him or her through to a cure.

As the disease progresses, however, its various effects show themselves. Muscle weakness moves to new parts of the body. Muscle cramps become more common and more severe in the arms, legs, chest, back, abdomen, jaw or throat. They are prolonged and very painful, sometimes leading to a tilting or stooping posture until they subside.

Even at rest, the muscles may be spastic; that is, they are tight and stiff, straightening the joints rather than contracting the joint, such as a stiff leg that will not relax to bend at the knee. Walking becomes affected; sleeping becomes difficult. It seems as if the muscles just will not cooperate. Patients and their caregivers spend a lot of time massaging, stretching, and heating the muscles.

Fatigue settles on the patient, as the surviving nerve cells increase their workload a hundredfold. The patient hesitates and gathers herself before climbing stairs. Lack of sleep and depression may add to fatigue.

For a host of reasons, sleep is interrupted starting in the early stages. This is a consistent complaint of patients. If it's not one thing, it's another: muscle contractions, spasticity, breathing difficulties, and a still-active mind consumed with anxiety, depression and the short future.

An embarrassing symptom of ALS is emotionality; patients tend to cry or laugh either spontaneously or as an over-reaction to difficult topics with emotional content. The emotional reaction may last for several minutes. The cause of this phenomenon is also probably muscular, due to the damage of muscles and their loss of the inhibiting function. Visitors to the patient may not understand that this effect, too, is a result of the disease.

In another embarrassing moment, the patient may drool. The normal, spontaneous swallowing which clears saliva from the mouth does not happen, and the facial muscles do not completely close the lips. The patient may also cough or gag due to the incomplete closure of the epiglottis while eating. This is a dangerous event due to the possibility of food getting into the larynx and lungs, which could result in pneumonia.

In this stage, as the physical realities and the prognosis become understood, a spiritual or philosophical response is developed which may differ from patient to patient. A certain kind of person sees the diagnosis as a call to war, or a personal challenge. With courage and determination – usually with a support system of family and friends – he or she goes into battle against the disease and searches the world for a cure or treatment. He or she may greet his or her local doctors' diagnosis and prognosis with skepticism and decide to find out for themselves. A variation on this finds the patient dealing mainly with symptoms as family and friends join the battle, not necessarily for a cure but for care.

Another kind of patient who lives near a major medical center and perhaps an ALS center puts his or her complete faith and fate in the hands of the specialists nearby. The patient is educated by his or her doctors, who monitor the progress of the disease and search for a clinical trial. The extent to which this patient becomes knowledgeable and avails himself or herself of the latest treatment options, or participates in clinical trials, depends on the activities of the local center. In the case of FALS families, a long-term relationship may already have been developed with the ALS center. The patient might be the second or third generation to be treated by the same doctors.

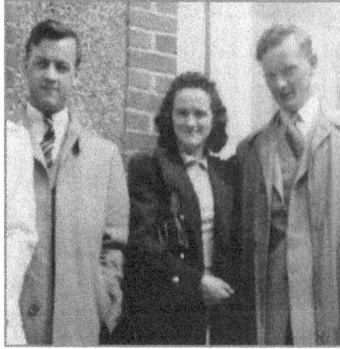

Clara and Forrest Langmaid (right)
with Forrest's brother Arnold (left).

CHAPTER 4

Tennie and Her Daughters

At the time that Tennie Mae Gaskill was born, 1894, familial ALS had been a recognized pattern of paralysis and early death within her family for almost sixty years. Tennie's grandfather was Wesley Ora Farr. He had died of the disease in 1891, just three years before Tennie was born. As a girl, Tennie may not have grown up with that tragic family history on her mind, but the facts were there, and Tennie would prove herself in her lifetime to be an inquisitive writer, genealogist and local historian. She would also contribute to the understanding in her time of ALS and especially of FALS.

Tennie Mae was born August 12, 1894 in Burke Hollow, Vermont. Her parents were Mary Matilda (Farr) and Tyler Gaskill. They lived on a farm in Burke Hollow, a little village between the two larger villages of the town – West Burke and East Burke. Tennie had two younger sisters, Marjoria and Laura. Tennie grew up to be a historian, writer and photographer, so her family today assumes that she was a good student. She attended the Burke Hollow School and graduated from Lyndon Institute in nearby Lyndon Center in the class of 1911 after having completed the business course. A memoir of the class of 1911 written by one of her classmates noted that it was a good thing that girls couldn't join the agriculture program because Tennie would have. After graduating from high school, she went immediately from being a student to being a teacher, teaching for one year in a little school near Chandler Pond in Lyndon. Her teaching career was interrupted by marriage.

At the age of nineteen, Tennie married Robert McGill. Robert was an itinerant blacksmith by trade, traveling to farms in the area to shoe horses, and also a small-time farmer. He was the brother of St. Johnsbury Fire Chief John McGill, and one of his blacksmith shops at one time was in St. Johnsbury. Tennie and Robert lived in several places, including Barnet and St. Johnsbury, as well as Monroe, New Hampshire. In 1920, they bought a small farm, along with a few animals and implements, on the North Danville Road, which goes from St. Johnsbury to the village of North Danville and then on to Danville.

Tennie's and Robert's childbearing started off sadly with two infant deaths, a boy who died at childbirth and a girl who lived only a year. They would eventually have seven healthy children who would live into adulthood. In 1936, when Tennie was forty-two and a mother of seven children, ages two through twenty-one, Robert was killed when kicked by a horse on the farm of George Nutter in Barnet. By that time, her daughters Viola and Rena were married, Williamina was nineteen and still living at home, as were the four youngest – Clara, Tyler, Robert and Calista. Tennie raised her children as a single mother for two years until she met Benjamin Toussaint, a North Danville man with three children of his own from a previous marriage.

Ben was born in Kingsley Falls, Quebec and grew up on a North Danville farm there. When he met Tennie, he was working, when he could get work, at the sawmill in North Danville village, and at Fairbanks Morse & Co. in St. Johnsbury where he was a scale packer in its box factory. The sawmill and box factory were part of one enterprise, the sawmill existing mainly to mill lumber from Fairbanks land for supply to Fairbanks Morse & Co, the large scale-making factory in St. Johnsbury. Local historians remember Ben as an accomplished and much sought-after dowser, someone who could find water (and all sorts of lost items) with a forked stick. Eventually, Tennie Toussaint—now having acquired the name by which she is still remembered—and Ben moved into the former North Danville 4H Camp on the road to St. Johnsbury. It was a modest dwelling, tucked in a tiny plot of land between the North Danville Road and the Sleepers River.

Marriage to Ben Toussaint brought Tennie and her children to the village of North Danville, which would become the family locus, and the setting for much of this story, for the next thirty-two years of Tennie's life. It remains a central place to the family. One of Tennie's grandchildren still lives there. As described by Tennie herself in an article written in 1955:

> There are some twenty-five homes, a Baptist Church, modern school building, general store, the town sheds, and a sawmill, situated right smack in the center of Caledonia County. Five spider-web roads lead out of the village past highly cultivated farms and to the summer homes of many city people, many of them artists and writers. The Sleepers River and its many tributaries drain this area, and the mill pond on the river above the dam is a favorite skating place in winter.

North Danville was a self-contained village in that era, with its own store, school, several churches, and a creamery. Dairy farming was the most prominent occupation; although for some it was also a sideline. Local sources who lived and farmed in the area have identified over thirty-five farm families producing milk in 1960 in the vicinity of North Danville alone, spaced along that web of roads leading out from the village. By 1960 the swift decline in the number of these small family farms was well underway, as bulk storage and transportation of milk replaced the ubiquitous 10-gallon milk cans that used to be brought to the creamery. The University of Vermont Center for Rural Studies estimates that Vermont farms in 1965 numbered approximately 6000. Today that figure is about 1026. Fewer but larger farms are the model today. Of the nine farms in the whole town of Danville today, seven are in North Danville. Three are still run by members of the Langmaid family who will appear later in our story.

Arlene Hubbard lived on one of the two farms whose barns were located right in the village, and she recalls a few other village features of the era. The general store was run by the E.T. & H.K. Ide Company, a grain and farm supply dealer. It was a full general store, with groceries and other sundries sold in the front and grain and farm supplies in the back. It was a village gathering place. Some men stopped by to play checkers, the children came for the penny candy, and farmers came for feed and farming hardware. For Tennie, it would have been a walk of about a mile one-way. Arlene's family pastured their cows outside of the village up the Old North Church Road where they had a small milking parlor. Their cows were herded through the village only in the spring and fall.

Tennie's granddaughters have described her as a "renaissance woman." She wrote articles for the local papers and historical journals, she took and collected photographs, and practiced a number of crafts, including knitting, caning chairs, gardening, canning, stenciling, and tole painting, the decorative art of painting on tin and other materials. She made an art form out of paintings made from photographs of local scenes. In March and April, she made maple syrup. Tennie sold most of her products to make extra money for the family.

Tennie never learned to drive and probably couldn't have afforded a car if she could drive. She walked from her home in North Danville to St. Johnsbury or Danville, or to other destinations in and around the village. A sight remembered by several family members and older residents of North Danville is of Tennie walking from her home to her sugarhouse on the other side of the village, a distance of two miles, perhaps carrying her lunch on the way to the sugarbush, and two open buckets of maple syrup on the way home.

Tennie's granddaughters have fond memories of her. They jumped at the chance to invite Tennie when the family was setting out on an errand by auto, and Tennie would drop everything to go along wherever they were headed. They also joined her at the sugarhouse. Her granddaughter Linda remembers being treated to eggs and hot dogs boiled in the sap.

Tennie's daughter Clara, who lost her father when she was fourteen, graduated from St. Johnsbury Academy at age fifteen and worked for a while in Woolworths Department Store in St. Johnsbury. In 1944, at age twenty-two, she married Forrest Langmaid. Forrest was twenty-seven and came from a family with long ties to the village. There were actually several farms in North Danville in his family. In the 1960's, Forrest's brother Hugh inherited the family farm on Coles Pond Road, his brother Arnold bought a farm outside the village on McDowell Road, while Forrest was eventually given his uncle Harry Drew's home in the village and the barn that sits right in the middle of the village. His brother Phil also bought a farm in Goss Hollow.

An outgoing man, whose asthma sometimes curtailed his work but rarely his talking, Forrest – or Fob, as most people knew him – was referred to as "the mayor of North Danville" and, his daughters say, was usually quite willing to stop work and talk. Driving through North Danville on a summer day during those years – as I did going to a summer job in 1966 – you might have encountered Fob in his barnyard on the main drag, talking with someone. According to Hollis Prior, Fob's son-in-law, Fob was also the defacto baby sitter and disciplinarian for the whole family. When little kids were getting under their parents' skin, they would say, "Go see Fob," and off to the barn the kids would go to be put to work (or dunked in the water trough as needed) by Forrest.

Clara's and Forrest's first child, Linda, was born in 1944, then four more children, so Clara was a busy mother for the next eighteen years. She became a 4H Leader, taught tap dancing at the Community Club, and sang in the church choir. A pretty, tiny woman, she was not involved very much in the hard work of farming. In fact, she carefully avoided it. As she told her daughters, "If you learn to do the milking, you'll find yourself in the barn doing the milking while your husband is off at the Caledonia County Fair."

Clara did enjoy one of the daily farm chores, however: going to get the cows at milking time. As her daughters got older, they had a choice in the late afternoon; they could either make the dinner or go get the cows. The Langmaid farm's cows grazed on fields that were a ways from the barn and separated from the barn by the paved road. The shortest route to fetch them was to bring them right down the middle of the village street, but over the years a safer route, and one probably more acceptable to their village neighbors, was established which brought them behind the school, across the road just to the west of town, then down along the river to the back of the barn. That chore Clara enjoyed, as the girls made supper. Eventually the three older girls—Linda, Mary, and Susan—were joined by brother, Cliff, born in 1955, and Jane, born in 1960.

An alto in the church choir, Clara sometime in February or March of 1962, missed a note and her voice began to sound different. At that time, it had been thirty years since a member of the family living in northeastern Vermont had suffered the symptoms of ALS. That was Tennie's uncle Frank Farr in Montpelier. The passage of time, and the family's collective amnesia had moved the disease, and its hereditary nature, off from the family's list of topics of awareness and conversation. Clara did not know what was happening to her. Apparently, when she did receive the diagnosis, she chose not to tell her children. "We just thought she was sick and would get better," her daughter Linda said.

The diagnosis was bulbar palsy. Clara's voice, breathing and swallowing deteriorated very sharply that spring and summer. Her mother Tennie, the family now believes, did know what was happening, that it was amyotrophic lateral sclerosis with the early symptom being bulbar palsy. Tennie had been researching the family history – probably for other reasons – and had come to some level of understanding of the sad and frightening history. Shocked and horrified, she kept it to herself for a while.

Clara received little treatment or modern care. Her case may have been recorded in the files at Massachusetts General Hospital but she never visited there. A small-town girl, her daughters explain, she didn't like the big hospital in Burlington where she was diagnosed, and she never returned there for treatment. Maybe she had been told that there was no treatment. She and Forrest went to a faith healer, the seventh-son-of-a-seventh-son, in Quebec. It is now believed that Clara had the family gene with the A4V mutation that results in the fast-developing form of the disease. From first symptoms to death, Clara lasted only nine months. The first cause of death listed on her death certificate was "Respiratory Failure"; the second cause "Progressive Bulbar Palsy."

If Clara Langmaid had contacted Massachusetts General Hospital or Mt. Sinai Hospital in New York (to see Lou Gehrig's doctors), or even the Mayo Clinic, there would not have been much they could have done for her. The section on ALS in the 1958 edition of *A Textbook of Clinical Neurology*, for instance, was written by Dr. Israel Wechsler, Gehrig's doctor. Written mostly in the first person ("I have seen") and citing only five sources in addition to two of his own papers, Wechsler offered little new in his sections on cause, pathology, symptoms, or diagnosis. In fact the scientific papers he cited were all published between 1906 and 1945, none in the subsequent thirteen years. "I have come to the conclusion that amyotrophic lateral sclerosis is not one disease entity but consists of at least three, possibly four, clinical syndromes of varying etiology," he wrote, anticipating some of the current thinking about variability in the disease. Wechsler, surveying his own patients, speculated that some were "subacute," others "chronic."

In the section on treatment, Wechsler sharply reduced his claims for vitamin treatment, writing that, "The vast majority of patients do not respond to Vitamin E therapy," but maintained that "I have seen a few who did." Overall, "The treatment in general is not satisfactory and is essentially palliative," he wrote. "The course is progressive with or without treatment, so that the prognosis is bad."

Also living in the village and able to help with Clara's care and take care of the children were Clara's sister Calista and her husband Charlie Myrick. Calista and Charlie had met in Georgia, where Charlie grew up, when Calista visited her brother Tyler who was stationed at Fort Benning. Tyler had married a Georgia girl, Martha Myrick, and it was Martha who introduced Calista to her brother Charlie. So brother and sister had married sister and brother. Charlie and Calista were married in 1954 and had moved back to Calista's hometown in 1955. Charlie eventually worked for Vermont Tap & Die in Lyndonville. By 1962, Charlie and Calista had three children – Steve, Dennis and John (a fourth son, Andrew, would be born in 1967, and a daughter, Cindy, would be born in 1971). When Clara got sick, Charlie and Calista, who lived across the street, offered to help. Charlie and his brother-in-law would regularly do the evening milking. Calista helped Forrest get the children off to school. Linda was a high school senior when her mother first began to develop symptoms. She and Mary, age sixteen, Susan, fourteen, Cliff, eight, and Jane, two, were living at home.

Linda worked in the White Mountains of New Hampshire that summer, and was alarmed as her mother got sicker and thinner. Nevertheless, when fall arrived, Linda enrolled in the nursing program at Fletcher Allen School of Nursing in Burlington. She went off to school still believing that her mother would recover. On October 18, 1962, Clara McGill Langmaid died at home. The head nurse at Fletcher Allen had the sad task of telling Linda. Her aunt came to Burlington to pick her up.

Soon, Clara's older sister Williamina, who was married and living in St. Johnsbury, also came to help with the children. Williamina had married a St. Johnsbury man in 1939, and they had one child, a boy who was in college. Each day, Williamina would drive out from St. Johnsbury to help Forrest with household tasks and watch over the two younger children.

In 1965, tragedy struck again. Williamina began to feel the fast-progressing symptoms of the disease herself—at first a weakness in one leg. She was treated for the leg problem, even undergoing an operation, but did not recover its use. Finally, she was diagnosed with ALS and had to retire from all duties. Before dying of the respiratory failure of ALS, however, she suffered a heart attack and died in 1966.

Tennie at some point—probably in the late 1940s—had apparently come to a full realization of the family history. In her lifetime, she had witnessed or heard of the young deaths of family members and the causes. Perhaps she was aware of her grandfather's young death at age fifty-three, three years before she was born; her mother's cousin Leon in 1906 at age thirty-seven down in Brattleboro; her mother's cousin Almira Stoddard in 1910; another cousin of her mother, Norman Farr in 1929; or her uncle Frank in 1932. Perhaps Frank's death at age sixty in Montpelier was the tipping point. It is hard to know; we can only imagine. Among the family archives is a three page typed list of Farr deaths that the family believes was Tennie's work. It is spotty and in places at odds with other records, but it may give us a clue as to her growing awareness as it lists deaths due to "paralysis, progressive muscular atrophy, palsy, and spinal sclerosis." The latest date on that list is 1906. One wonders: did Tennie follow the illness and death of Lou Gehrig in 1941?

However she came to it, Tennie apparently faced a dilemma: the family disease must either be confronted or hidden. She may have decided in a way to do both: sharing the facts with doctors but hiding them from the family. Interviews with Tennie's grandchildren suggest that when Tennie's daughter Clara got sick in the spring of 1962, Tennie allowed the family to believe that Clara might get well, and that her disease was a sporadic event, not part of any family pattern of inheritance.

On a winter day in 1963, Charlie was in Tennie's home when he saw Tennie put some papers and file folders in the woodstove. He didn't know what he was seeing at the time, but soon after Calista informed him: Tennie had burned her research on the family disease. It has always been Charlie's understanding that Tennie had stumbled upon the family pattern in the process of doing basic genealogy, and that she came to the task without any inkling of what she would find. The story is told in the family that way: that Tennie had discovered the pattern of deaths in her family from paralysis and palsy, she had been horrified, but she kept it to herself. Then she had watched her own daughter suffer and die over a brief nine-month span, and the tragic heredity had been confirmed.

It was also Charlie's understanding that Tennie was concerned about her daughter Viola and what she would do with the information. Viola had moved to Georgia, and like her mother, she was interested in family history. Viola had begun to ask her mother questions about the family disease, and had possibly even been in touch with researchers at Emory University in Georgia. Perhaps to simply protect her family living in Vermont from the truth for as long as she could, Tennie had burned her copies of the charts and notes she had compiled.

Apparently, however, Tennie at the time that she burned all copies of the notes had already shared her family history with doctors. In the 1951 article mentioned in Chapter Two in which Dr. Madeleine Brown of Boston's Massachusetts General Hospital identified two families afflicted with familial ALS, she gave credit to Tennie for aiding her in her research. Somehow, Tennie had come to understand years before her own daughters got sick that medical scientists were studying what would become known as familial amyotrophic lateral sclerosis (FALS). Researchers would focus on the Farr family, and their research required establishing relations with some members of the family. Who contacted whom first, or how Dr. Brown of Massachusetts General Hospital learned of the Farrs in northern Vermont, or how Tennie learned of Dr. Brown's research, is not known. Tennie's notes, in any case, found their way into Dr. Brown's files and have recently been shared with the family.

Looking at the family pattern, and knowing what we do about

Tennie, we can calculate and imagine what she knew of the family history before her own daughter's death. She must have known a lot. There were just too many people around her, many living in northern Vermont, who had died young of the disease, their death certificates listing paralysis, palsy, respiratory failure and other symptoms, and too many people who would have known them. Plus, we know that she was curious and realistic. Nevertheless, there seems to have been a pattern of avoiding the subject, out of a desire to protect others, especially the younger generation. Many members of the family have told me as much. "We just didn't talk about it," they say. This pattern of some members of the family knowing a lot and others being kept in the dark would result in several instances of surprise and shock as new victims would begin to develop symptoms in years to come. Also, family members living in distant parts of the country would not learn of others' diagnosis.

. . . . .

While the Farr family was dealing with the illnesses of first Clara and then her sister Williamina in Vermont in the early sixties, away from major medical centers, the newspapers contained the story of another nationally-known figure: Henry A. Wallace, the 33rd Vice-President of the United States. In June of 1964, then retired at age seventy-five and living on his estate in South Salem, New York, Wallace noticed a sharp deterioration in his tennis game. His left foot seemed to drag. Wallace had always been a very active man, and even at seventy-five had usually run a half-mile and did twenty-two pushups a day. He was also a man with a wide-ranging, scientific mind and was a voracious reader with a lot of interests.

In August, doctors at the hospital in Danbury, Connecticut, according to Wallace's own account, "gave me the myelogram with olive oil and iodine [a radiographic picture of the spinal cord], the electromyogram [a graphic look at the electric current of muscular action], brain scan with mercury 203, and various tests to eliminate diabetes." "Finally," he wrote, "they decided on amyotrophic lateral sclerosis, or ALS." Wallace went to the Mayo Clinic in November, where the diagnosis was confirmed, and eventually to the National Institute of Health in Bethesda, Maryland. It was at NIH that Wallace began to write a fifteen-page piece entitled "Reflections of an ALSer" quoted above. Wallace wanted to play an active role in figuring out what was wrong with him, and also had the best of medical care available to him. His essay gives us an excellent snapshot of the causal theories and treatment ideas of the mid-1960s, and it seems that Wallace and his doctors would try anything.

Henry Agard Wallace came from a famous family of Iowa, mostly associated with agriculture. His grandfather, the first Henry Wallace, started *Wallace's Farmer* in 1896, which would become an influential journal of news, opinion, and policy discussions in the Corn Belt. His father, Henry C. Wallace, carried on the family's influential tradition and served as Warren Harding's Secretary of Agriculture. As a teenager in the first decade of the twentieth century, Henry A. Wallace had taken an interest in hybrid corn, believing that the current varieties of corn were good looking but not necessarily high yielding. This interest would eventually lead to him perfecting a high-yield corn brand and starting the Pioneer Hi-Bred Company, which would eventually make him and his heirs very wealthy.

Following his father into politics (although switching parties) Henry A. Wallace served as Franklin Roosevelt's Secretary of Agriculture for two terms, then as FDR's Vice President in his third term from 1940-1944. Roosevelt had named Wallace Commerce Secretary during his fourth term, and Truman at first kept him in that position as the last of the New Deal leaders in the cabinet. In that position, Wallace continued to push for progressive policies and also for peace as the country veered to the right. Truman fired Wallace as Secretary of Commerce over their differences in September of 1946.

Henry A. Wallace's last campaign was a tumultuous and controversial run for President as a candidate of the Progressive Party in the 1948 election, in which he garnered only 2.4 percent of the popular vote, and no electoral votes. He retired from public life in 1950 at sixty-two, and returned to being a full-time farmer. He and his wife Ilo, rather than returning to Iowa, had purchased a 115-acre farm in Westchester County, NY, overlooking the Connecticut ridges. They had named the farm Farvue, and there they settled.

Rules of the Federal Food and Drug Administration were revised in 1962 to require drug manufacturers to prove that a drug was not only safe but effective. This would soon lead to the current system of double-blind drug trials required before FDA approval. However in 1964, as Henry A. Wallace and his doctors discussed treatment, there seems to have been no restrictions and little protocol. They would try anything for a while to see if there was any effect. Wallace writes in "Reflections" that he understood something of the process of de-myelinization: the deterioration and loss of the myelin sheath that protects the nerve fibers in the spinal cord. "I began to wonder about slowing down the process of de-myelinization," he wrote, "and of even restoring the myelin."

Wallace's bulbar muscles had begun to weaken, and he gave his last public talk in October of 1964. Wallace and his Connecticut doctors tried a substance called Wobe, which he referred to as "a proteolytic enzyme mixture," for six months, with no effect. Then they tried the dried sicca cells of Niehans, and injections of H3 procaine.

It wasn't until late September of 1965 that Wallace entered the National Institutes of Health in Bethesda, Maryland. His ability to swallow had deteriorated markedly, so physicians at NIH first inserted a feeding tube in his trachea. Wallace apparently began his journal at that time and began to list the treatments tried by NIH physicians: glandular extracts from the stomach, liver and pancreas of his own body; bone marrow (at Wallace's own suggestion); intra-muscular injections; and palliative medicines such as atropine and bella donna.

"I look upon myself as an ALS guinea pig," he wrote, "willing to try out almost anything." Wallace took a great interest in the disease as his NIH doctors continued to give him much hope.

He discussed with his doctors the latest developments and theories regarding the disease, including the high incidence of ALS among the natives of Guam, the statistics of the disease in the US, and the range in the duration of the disease from patient to patient.

Wallace was philosophical about the disease and recorded his feelings and observations in familiar terms:

> *Truly, ALS is a unique experience. There is no pain. Apparently your eyes and brain are not affected. Therefore, you can calmly watch the rest of your body slowly disintegrate, moving from the left leg to certain muscles in the left arm. Then, no muscles in the cheeks, very few in the tongue and throat . . .*
>
> *After a year of ALS, you begin to feel a little like a disembodied spirit in purgatory. Of course, you come back to this earth with a bump when you try to walk or talk or eat.*
>
> *The amazing thing is how many people come to see you. Different people have different attitudes in calling on sick people. A great many bring books for you to read. Apparently, the idea is to give you more handles to this world so that you will not slip away for lack of interest.*
>
> *ALS gives you a ringside seat at your own dissolution. With a clear mind, you can consider life and death and the eternal verities.*
>
> *This ALSer has had a rich experience with the goodness of man as exhibited toward those who are unfortunate.*

On October 28, Wallace returned to Farvue by ambulance, and finished his essay there. He ended his "Reflections," with the date of

November 1965. In its last paragraph he listed some of his remaining goals, still on his agenda even though he had very little time left. "I do want to play my part in developing a superior brown-egg chicken," he wrote or dictated, "a strawberry with a unique flavor, and a fine type of miniature gladiolus. I have written a letter to President Johnson on the importance of decentralization – my last effort to influence contemporary affairs."

Henry A. Wallace died of respiratory failure in Danbury Hospital on November 18, 1965. From first symptoms until his death, he had lived fifteen months.

· · · · ·

Tennie May Gaskill McGill Toussaint died on August 23, 1973 at the age of seventy-nine, probably of ALS. I write *probably* because the family does not fully agree. "I think she wanted to die of ALS," said her granddaughter Linda Vance. It would all make sense—a kind of poetic justice—for her to suffer the same fate as her children and all of those in the family whom she had researched. Tennie died, said Linda, before she showed any definite symptoms of ALS. Linda remembers being four-months pregnant with her son Curtis in March of 1973, and visiting Tennie at her sugarhouse off the Old North Church Road in North Danville. Tennie would have walked there from her home on the North Danville Road, often cutting across lots through the snow rather than taking the indirect route by the roads. Tennie was doing the hard work of sugaring – lugging sap, feeding the arch with chunks of hardwood, drawing off the syrup into three-gallon buckets – and Linda remembers admiring her for her strength and spirit at age seventy-nine. Tennie hardly showed the signs of someone afflicted with a disease that causes muscle wasting.

When she declined suddenly, Linda reasons, she told her doctors about the family history, and they obliged her later by listing her cause of death as "familial muscular atrophy." What difference did it make to the doctors? That is what Linda figures. Tennie's daughter-in-law

Irma, Robert's wife, who also lived in the village, kept a journal in which she recorded that Tennie died of a stroke. That was what was told to members of the family not living in the area.

But Tennie's son-in-law Charlie Myrick sees it differently. That spring and summer, Charlie and his wife Calista were looking after Tennie. Charlie remembers the sugaring, but he also remembers that it was right about that time that Tennie began to experience weakness in her right leg. He also remembers that she traveled with them by car to Georgia for the funeral of Charlie's sister Martha, who was married to Tennie's son Tyler. Martha died on May 3, 1973 a month after the sugaring season. It was a difficult trip; walking was difficult for Tennie, as was travel in the car. Charlie recalls that he, Calista and Tennie made an unplanned stop on the way home and took a motel room because Tennie was in so much discomfort riding in the car. She could barely walk by the time they got home.

When she got home, Tennie visited Dr. Elbridge Johnston, her regular doctor. Dr. Johnston, Charlie recalls, was stumped by Tennie's symptoms. Then Tennie told him about the family history and gave her symptoms a name. Dr. Johnston said he would look into it in his medical textbooks. When he did, he made the diagnosis of familial amyotrophic lateral sclerosis. As the disease progressed, Tennie lost the use of her legs, and her left arm. She was breathing with difficulty. It seems to Charlie in retrospect that her voice muscles must have deteriorated before her actual breathing muscles; she talked only in a whisper. In retrospect, Tennie's quick decline from strong and fit farm woman to a barely walking patient can be explained by the A4V mutation, as all Farrs will have the fast-progressing form of the disease.

Tennie was in and out of the hospital that summer. Eventually, however, she was brought to the home of Charlie and Calista, where she died. The cause of death reported on her death certificate by Dr. Maurice Rowe: familial muscular atrophy.

By the time of Tennie Toussaint's death in 1973, three of her children and their families were still living in Vermont. Calista and

Charlie Myrick and their four children lived in North Danville, as did Robert and his wife Irma and their three children. Rena and her husband Gerald Longchamps, with three children, had settled in Tennie's hometown of Burke Hollow, not far away.

By 1973 there was a Georgia contingent. Viola had moved to Georgia with her husband Errol Ralston and they had had six children. Their youngest, Janet, had been born in 1960. Viola came north in 1973 to be with her mother. She stayed with Calista and Charlie and agreed with them that Tennie's symptoms were those of ALS. Viola had remained interested in learning as much as she could about the family disease and would become active in the Georgia chapter of the ALS Association. Tyler McGill had married Charlie Myrick's sister Martha in 1946, and they had moved to Georgia with their five children, the youngest of whom had been born in 1967.

As for the next generation in Danville, Tennie's grandchildren, in 1973 all of Clara and Forrest Langmaid's children were living in Danville or North Danville. Linda had married Roy Vance in 1963, and by 1973 they had four children. They had lost a son, Charles, to crib death in 1972. The fourth son, Curtis, was born in August of 1973, five days before his grandmother's death. They would have two more sons. Mary had married Hollis Prior in 1968, and by 1973 they had three children. Susan and her husband Dwayne Lynaugh were married in 1970. They would have two children, born in 1975 and 1981. Clif was eighteen years old in 1973 and working with his father on the family farm. Jane, the youngest of Clara's and Forrest's children, was thirteen years old in 1973. Susan and Dwayne lived in North Danville village, while Linda and Roy and Mary and Hollis lived in Danville.

Williamina's husband Howard lived in St. Johnsbury in 1973. Calista and her husband Charlie had settled in a house on the North Danville Road, which runs from St. Johnsbury to North Danville village. They raised five children, all of whom attended the Danville schools. In 1973, their oldest son Steve was sixteen, Dennis was fifteen, John thirteen, Andrew seven, and Cindy two. Tennie's son Robert and his wife Irma had three children by 1973. They too lived on the North Danville Road. In that year, their daughter Melinda was eighteen, son Robert seventeen, and Douglas twelve.

By 1973 when Tennie died, the children and grandchildren of Clara and Williamina knew—or could have known—that their mothers had inherited the defective gene that triggers ALS, but Viola, Rena, Tyler, Calista, Robert and their children could all hope that they did not have the gene. In 1973, Viola turned fifty-eight, Rena fifty-five, Tyler fifty, Robert forty-four, and Calista thirty-nine. They were all in the stage of life at which ALS normally strikes. They may have disagreed about whether their mother had died of ALS, but they couldn't escape the fact that she had carried the gene, having passed it on to two of her daughters.

For the next twenty-five years, ALS did not haunt the members of the Farr family living in northern Vermont. The Vermont Farrs were able to put the disease out of their everyday thoughts. This was so even though their aunt Rena, another daughter of Tennie, died quietly in a nursing home in St. Johnsbury in 1988 at age seventy with symptoms of ALS, and they were made aware of the death also in 1988 of a cousin, age forty-eight, in Georgia.

PART III

The Modern Era
(1974 – 1999)

The Disease Progresses

Sleep becomes a problem fairly early for many ALS patients. Lying down, the patient loses the help from gravity, which in a standing or a sitting position, acts to push the abdominal contents down, helping the diaphragm, which is the muscular group used in inhalation. Patients try several things to get comfortable, such as lying on their side, propping themselves up with pillows, or sleeping in a recliner. Before long, patients may seek the help of a noninvasive breathing mask to force air into their lungs.

Most patients lose weight, due to difficulties of eating or appetite and attitude. Patients are urged by their doctors to try to keep up their weight, which also means to keep up their nutritional intake. Fatigue is also a common problem fairly early, and again it may have physiological or psychological causes.

Visitors to a patient may also notice musculoskeletal signs, such as foot or hand deformities, a claw-like hand, or sagging shoulders. Muscles contract or shorten abnormally and can be very painful. This results in a vicious circle as the pain makes the patient reluctant to use the joint, then the muscles atrophy further. Caregivers and professionals provide sometimes aggressive physical therapy and range of motion exercises to forestall the worst of these effects.

ALS patients almost always end up in a wheelchair. Before that, however, they may walk with a noticeable lean or limp, then use a cane, a walker, perhaps a shopping cart, or walk with assistance. They may for a while be able to use the muscles of the hip and knee joint but may develop a *foot drop* in which they are unable to hold up their toes in a stride and their toes hit the floor before their heels. Some patients even use a spring device from ankle to toe to hold up the toe. One side of the body is usually weaker sooner than the other.

Eventually, patients come to live in some sort of a hospital chair or recliner. They spend both day and night in the chair. Both urinary urgency and/or constipation seem to accompany the disease in these middle stages. When they can't get out of the chair, even with assistance, they use a catheter for the release of urine. Regularity in bowel movement becomes a struggle as the patient and his or her caregivers try to maintain hydration, some activity, fiber intake, and medicine intake. The muscles of the bowels atrophy. Constipation and diarrhea are constant worries. "Dignity disappears and you are very happy to get a clean pair of pajamas," wrote Henry A. Wallace.

Due to immobility, the hands and feet may swell. The legs need to be elevated. The patient may wear elastic stockings to keep the swelling down.

For a patient in a loving relationship, sex becomes both a blessing and a problem. The ability to have sex is not at first a problem for male ALS patients; they can get an erection. The problem for both men and women patients is with other usually voluntary muscles, which may contract involuntarily in the sex act. They may cramp or twitch or cause discomfort. A loving couple with desires, however, can work together to find positions which make it possible. Also, of course, it is good therapy.

Speech becomes slurred and slow. Swallowing becomes difficult. Patients often opt eventually for a feeding tube. At first, it may be used only for extra nutrition while the pleasures of eating can be obtained by eating small amounts slowly. Eventually, however, many patients opt for either a nasal tube, a percutaneous endoscopic gastrostomy (PEG) stomach tube, or a percutaneous endoscopic jejunostomy (PEJ) tube, also in the stomach. It is a crucial decision point for patients, as they decide whether to prolong their lives through this artificial and invasive means.

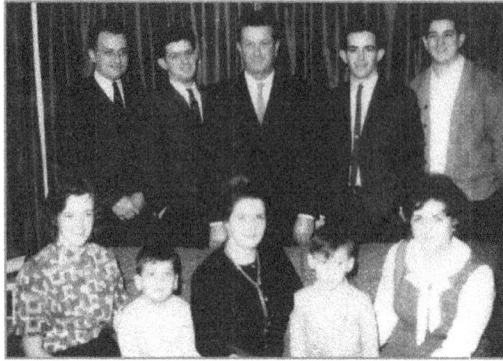

Viola Ralston (seated middle) and her family. Seated L to R: daughter Janet, Janet's son Brett, Viola, Janet's son Scott, and daughter Brenda. Standing L to R: son Bob, son Kenneth, husband Errol, son Keith and son Kelly.

CHAPTER 5

Kelly and Rena

Kelly Ralston was a lineman for Southern Bell Telephone in June of 1987. He was forty-two years old, a father of three. He and his wife Joanna lived in McDonough, Georgia. The previous winter he had fallen from a pole, and then he began to feel a weakness in his legs. At first he thought that he had a pinched nerve as a result of the fall. He went to a chiropractor. He didn't tell his mother Viola at first, probably not wanting to worry her and perhaps not wanting to accept that his muscle weakness might be a symptom of ALS.

Kelly's mother Viola, Tennie Toussaint's oldest child, had moved to Georgia with her husband Errol Ralston. Errol was a Vermont man too, but the couple was drawn to the south by the warmer climate, plus Viola's brother Tyler lived there. By 1987, Viola Ralston was running the Georgia chapter of the ALS Association out of her home. She was a volunteer, an activist, and a home aide for patients with ALS. She worked closely with doctors at Emory University Hospital.

Her son had moved from New Jersey to Georgia at his mother's urging, and had found a good job with the telephone company in 1966. In Georgia, his first marriage had ended and he eventually met and married another Southern Bell employee, Joanna Lee. Joanna and Kelly had added a third child to their family, and had moved from an Atlanta suburb to McDonough, near his mother and siblings. They were a tight family. At age forty-two, Kelly was still working a demanding, physical job, and was known for his strength and vitality. He was gregarious and fun, his family recalls, and loved his family and neighborhood. He had been baptized in 1969 after meeting Joanna, but he was not a regular church-goer.

The first symptom that Joanna recalls, suggesting that something was wrong with Kelly, was a sore neck, but then he felt a general weakness and began to have trouble doing his job. Early in 1988, he resigned from his job. Kelly told his mother that he was feeling a pronounced weakness in his legs. Viola then experienced what she had dreaded, and the grim, inexorable progress of the disease that awaited Kelly would have been laid out in her mind. She suggested that Kelly contact neurologists at Emory with whom she was familiar.

Kelly did contact Emory, went in for tests, and was diagnosed with ALS. He and the southern branch of the Farr family then were entered into the FALS database. Even though their mother was active in the Georgia Chapter of the ALS association, the children of Viola Ralston and their families were not fully aware of the family history. "It was not that we were uneducated about it," Kelly's wife recalls, "but we were ignorant still." Joanna had known something of the family history when she married Kelly, but she had not lived with the thought that it could actually happen to them. Scott Ralston, Kelly's nephew and Viola's grandson, in fact, hearing of his uncle's symptoms, wanted to learn more about ALS so he called the Georgia chapter of the ALS Association. His grandmother answered. Thinking that he had dialed the wrong number, he tried it again, and his grandmother answered again. The ALS Association Georgia chapter was in her home.

Kelly Ralston had the fast-developing form of ALS and his weakness progressed rapidly. Becoming more a man of faith, he put himself in God's hands and accepted his fate. He was "going to a better place," he is remembered saying. For most of the year as an ALS patient, he chose not to take any extraordinary measures, including help with his breathing. In his last weeks and months, he wanted to spend time with family and friends. He also wanted to know and speak the truth about the disease, Joanna recalls, not wanting to dwell in false hope or myth. He embraced his faith, holding Bible studies in his home. His friends stayed with him until the end, frequently visiting and building him a ramp when he graduated to a motorized chair. Kelly did not revisit Emory University for treatment or clinical trials. In his case, the paralysis of the disease spread rapidly, and by summer he was bedridden. Toward the end, he was getting a little help with breathing through an apparatus.

Before long, Kelly was in respiratory distress. On the day that he died, November 3, 1988, a number of people, including family, friends, his minister, and his doctor, were in the room. As his daughter Cindy remembers his last moments, he went into a sort of coma, losing consciousness, then opened his eyes one last time and spoke, indicating that he had seen his savior. His last word was "Jesus."

The Vermont members of the Farr family were notified of Kelly's passing and of his funeral, but no one from Vermont could get away to attend the service in Georgia. This further widened a gap between the northern and southern Farrs. In the twenty-seven years since, there has been little contact between the two branches, a fact about which both sides feel regret. Brenda Peterson, Kelly's sister, remembers with fondness her visits to Vermont: her time with her grandmother Tennie and Ben, hanging around Fob's barn, playing with all her Vermont cousins. They attribute the lack of contact to the size of the family (Tennie had seven children and twenty-seven grandchildren), to distance in the era before email and social media, to career demands, and to small slights and cultural differences. It also may be true that during this era grandma

Tennie's apparent plan to keep the burden of heredity off the shoulders of her family worked. Their common experience of ALS, which might have brought them together, instead kept them apart. "We just didn't talk about it," they say.

Rena Longchamps was another of Tennie's daughters. She grew up in Barnet and North Danville, Vermont, and married Gerald Longchamps when she was seventeen in 1935. Rena and Gerald soon bought a motel and restaurant in Franconia, New Hampshire which they ran until 1963, when they sold it and bought the Gaskill farm, Tennie's girlhood home in Burke Hollow. The property consisted of sixth-four acres, a two-story colonial house with a CONDEMNED sign on it, and a tumbling down barn. According to her grandson Chuck, Rena and Gerald jacked up the house to replace the foundation and saved the old homestead. Gerald was a skilled carpenter, which became his career when they moved back to Vermont. Rena lived on the Gaskill place for the next twenty-five years. Her grandson Chuck lives there now.

Rena and Gerald had their first child, daughter Rena Bessie who came to be called Betty, soon after their marriage. They eventually adopted two sons--David and Russell Lee--through Catholic Charities. In 1957, daughter Betty, at age seventeen, gave birth to a boy whom she named Charles. Rena and Gerald decided to bring him up as their son and legally adopted him. Charles, known as Chuck, grew up thinking that his grandmother was his mother, and that his mother was his sister. He didn't learn the truth about his parentage until he was a grown man and one of his brothers let it slip. Betty would eventually have four more children. She and her first husband had a boy and a girl, and she and her second husband, Michael Jablonski, had two children, a boy and a girl. Eventually, she and Michael adopted Betty's first two children. They offered to adopt Chuck, but he was a grown man in his forties and declined.

Rena had survived two bouts with cancer, including surgeries, and the family had always feared that cancer would be the cause of her death, but early in the winter of 1988, at age sixty-nine she began to feel muscle weakness in her left foot. Before long she was using a walker, and then was in a chair, unable to walk. Eventually, she could not be cared for at home and was admitted to the St. Johnsbury Health and Rehabilitation Center, a nursing home. She received little of the palliative care, including breathing aids, which was available to patients at that time. She was not treated by a neurologist, and did not visit any major medical center in Boston, Burlington or Hanover. Toward the end, Chuck remembers, she could use her hand and fingers to push the buttons of a cassette tape player, but could not use her arm to turn over a cassette. Rena was visited regularly by her family. She passed away of respiratory failure in August of 1988. She was seventy years old. Her death certificate records that from onset of symptoms to death the time period was nine months, her death "due to or as a consequence of – peripheral motor neuropathy."

Given the history of FALS in her family, the symptoms that Chuck observed, and the wording of the cause of death on her death certificate, Chuck is today convinced that she was another victim of the family disease. For him, it all adds up: the muscle wasting, the progression of the disease, and the immediate cause of death as noted on the death certificate: respiratory arrest. In an interview twenty-six years after the fact, her doctor, Dr. John Ajamie said that he could not recall the particulars of Rena's illness, and the records have been destroyed. He also was not aware even now that Rena was a member of the Farr family with a long history of ALS. Learning that, however, and being reminded of the wording on the death certificate which he had completed, Dr. Ajamie stated that her symptoms, labeled as "peripheral motor neuropathy," were consistent with ALS.

Rena was never diagnosed by a neurologist, however, never visited a major medical center, and failed very quickly. She had a history of other medical problems and symptoms that included difficulty in the use of one arm. She was seventy years old, past the usual age of onset. For these reasons, her nieces, Linda Vance and Susan Lynaugh, the two people most familiar with the family history and the symptoms of ALS, are unconvinced that their aunt died of ALS. They don't remember anyone suggesting it at the time of her illness. And besides, the cause of death as penciled by Dr. Ajamie, is peripheral motor neuropathy, not familial muscular atrophy (their mother's listed cause of death), and definitely not amyotrophic lateral sclerosis.

As they argued about their grandmother Tennie, they now argue that the family history, and the fear of ALS, is driving the retrospective diagnosis. For all members of the Farr family, ALS is a specter; it is always there, crowding into their thinking. Driven by that fear, they reason, Rena probably thought to herself: This is it, it is my turn. As the doctor did with Tennie, they reason, so did Rena's doctor. He went along; he took his cues from the family.

If Rena did die from FALS, that would mean that of Tennie's seven children, three daughters died of ALS and two, Viola and Calista, were carriers of the toxic gene. Tennie's two sons and their children and grandchildren apparently did not inherit the gene. Son Tyler died in 1979 from a stroke, and son Robert, age eighty-six, was living without ALS symptoms in the spring of 2015 in the same St. Johnsbury nursing home where his sister had been living at the time of her death in 1988.

Rena's son Chuck, upon learning in his forties that his adoptive mother was actually his grandmother, learned that his own chances of having that gene mutation went from fifty percent to twenty-five percent. He lives today with the thought that, while he is in the genetic line and believes that his grandmother died of the disease, his mother did not. Betty lived to be seventy-three and died of respiratory failure from smoking. His two adoptive brothers are of course not in the genetic line, but Betty's other four children are, and to date the disease has not appeared among Chuck's half-sisters or half-brother.

· · · · ·

Families with a history of ALS have been the most important clusters or data sets of patients for researchers studying the causes of ALS. Although familial clusters of ALS patients make up only about ten per cent of all patients, their disease has all of the same characteristics as sporadic ALS, and, it has been assumed, has the same cause or set of causes. Researchers have believed that if they focus on familial ALS (FALS) patients and their family members, they may be able to locate the gene—or actually the gene defect— that they have in common, and from there perhaps they will trace the pathways of the disease. Then they can begin to look for ways to block those pathways or to turn off the defective gene, sometimes also referred to as the gene mutation or a "toxic" gene.

The researcher whose team is credited with finding the first gene associated with FALS is Dr. Robert H. Brown Jr. of the University of Massachusetts Medical School in Worcester, MA. At a panel discussion in November of 2001 as part of a meeting of the Amyotrophic Lateral Sclerosis/Motor Neuron Disease (ALS/MND) Association, Dr. Brown explained to the mixed audience the enormous contribution of families in the search for the defective gene. He used the Farrs as his representative family, noting that they had been in the medical literature for over 100 years.

As a slide of the Farr family genealogy was projected on the screen with its female circles and male squares indicating those who were affected and not affected by the disease, Dr. Brown pointed out the generation of Samuel Farr, and at the bottom of the screen his great grandchildren. "Three out of five [of the great grandchildren] have developed ALS and died before the age of forty," he explained. "So obviously this is a terrible signature of a very, very bad gene defect."

"Now as you know, the one saving grace from a pedigree like this is you can move from this to find genes, and it was indeed this kind of family that helped our consortium—myself, Teepu Siddique, Peggy Vance, Jonathan Haines, and many others—find the first ALS gene in 1993."

Today it is possible for a member of a FALS family to provide licensed labs a sample of his or her DNA and learn whether he or she has the defective gene, but before the revolution in genetic studies and genetic medicine, the only way for a person to determine whether he or she might have the defective gene was simply to observe the pattern of the disease in the family. That process in the case of ALS—and the Farrs—started with the paper by Dr. Osler in 1880, and was apparently resumed in the 1940s with the work of Dr. Madelaine Brown at Massachusetts General Hospital, as described in Chapter 1.

It seems that Dr. Madelaine Brown's work did lead to Dr. Robert H. Brown's work at Mass General. Today, the keeper of the family trees is Diane McKenna-Yasek, a nurse on Dr. Robert Brown's team at UMass Medical School. McKenna-Yasek was on the staff of Dr. Brown at MGH before moving with him to UMass in 2008. When I interviewed her in August of 2012, she pulled out a set of charts which Dr. Madelaine Brown used to use to illustrate her talks about ALS and heredity, then showed me her own computer screen of branches and branches of the Farr family all over the country showing family members represented as squares and circles. The circles and squares of those who died of, or were affected by, the disease were filled in.

Robert H. Brown Jr. grew up in Maryland. After graduating from Amherst College in 1969, he received a PhD from Oxford University and his MD from Harvard University. He joined the staff of Mass General in 1979. He has said that he first took an interest in "the genetic underpinnings" of ALS when he diagnosed and treated Oscar Horvitz, a Chicago accountant whose son was a scientist at MIT. Mr. Horvitz died of ALS in 1989. Dr. Brown and Oscar Horvitz's son, H. Robert Horvitz, embarked on a collaborative study of ALS in the emerging field of human genetics. Robert Horvitz would go on to win the Nobel Prize for Medicine in 2002 for his work in understanding cell death or apoptosis.

Dr. Brown's team used a simple but time-consuming process to find FALS families and put together a comprehensive database of patients and their families. They wrote letters to neurologists all over the world, asking for help locating families who had suffered multi-generational ALS. By the late 1980s, they had collaborators from the U.S., Canada, England, Scotland, Belgium, France, Israel, Sweden, and Saudi Arabia. In fact, Dr. Brown told a gathering at Amherst College in 2008, it was a large family in Belgium that had led him and his team to the discovery of the defective gene.

In 1991, Dr. Brown wrote a "progress report" on his team's study of gene linkage and ALS. His team had enrolled 106 families by 1989, he reported. The team's charts and databases represented 3,200 individuals, 124 of whom were affected at the time of publication. He and his team had identified three clinical subsets of FALS: 1) typical autosomal dominant type, 2) atypical long surviving type, and 3) a benign juvenile form of the disease found in Tunisia. He argued in the progress report that such a study could lead to: A) a better understanding of sporadic ALS also, since the clinical findings in the familial and sporadic forms were indistinguishable; B) identification of the protein responsible for the disease; and C) new directions in research in all forms of motor neuron disease. Initial gene linkage probes had excluded linkage at forty seven loci, with "weakly positive" linkages on three chromosomes.

In another progress report published in May of 1991, Dr. Brown and his group reported linkage to chromosome 21. Using a computer program to calculate the odds, the group came up with a score which expressed the likelihood of linkage between a particular chromosome and the disease. DNA had been obtained from FALS patients in several forms, including whole blood and frozen autopsy tissue.

The breakthrough in the search for a genetic cause of FALS finally occurred in 1993. Dr. Brown and his team reported in the journal *Nature* that they had established "tight genetic linkage" between FALS and a particular enzyme: Cu/Zn superoxide dismutase. The defective gene has henceforth been known to family members and the profession as SOD1. SOD1, the team reported, is a "homodimeric metalloenzyme that catalyzes the dismutation of the toxic superoxide anion O_2 to O_2 and H_2O_2." Patient guides explain it this way: the gene coordinates the manufacture of a specific protein (superoxide dismutase) whose function is to clean the cell of waste products of cell metabolism. Those waste products are known as oxygen free radicals. The SOD1 normally functions as an antioxidant, helping to clean the cells, but the defective gene instead produces a toxic protein that damages them. "We believe the simplest hypothesis is that mutations we have identified in the SOD1 gene cause FALS," they wrote. As Dr. Brown explained it later in the 2001 meeting, SOD1 is a very abundant protein in the body, and works in a crucial way all over the body by binding copper and zinc, and by "soaping up or sopping up" and in some way "metabolizing" free radicals.

In their paper, the authors offered several hypotheses to explain the damaging process, including alternative ideas that the SOD1 activity might be too reduced, or that it might be too increased: underworking or overworking. Also to be explained by further research: how this process actually damages specific motor neurons so that they don't do their job of stimulating the muscles.

The authors concluded their 1993 paper with one hopeful paragraph about therapy. "If indeed toxicity caused by oxygen free radicals is the primary pathogenetic mechanism for motor neuron death in FALS and perhaps in sporadic ALS as well," they wrote, "measures that diminish this toxicity might blunt the devastating course of the disease. Clinical trials of either SOD itself or compounds that penetrate the central nervous system and decrease levels of free radicals should be feasible."

The watershed 1993 paper listed as co-authors, in addition to Robert H. Brown Jr. then of Massachusetts General Hospital, Daniel H. Rosen of MGH, Teepu Siddique of Northwestern University, Diane McKenna-Yasek, and H. Robert Horvitz, among thirty-three scientists from all over the world.

The discovery of the SOD1 gene defect has meant a lot to the Farrs and other FALS families. It has given them hope, for one thing, that treatments could be developed, and that they may be developed this time based on theories that got to the genetic heart of the problem. Treatments for ALS would be based on an understanding of cell death and the true pathways of the disease.

The SOD1 discovery also clarified the Farr family's exact pattern of inheritance as autosomal dominant. *Autosomal* means that it is equally likely that a female or a male would inherit the gene mutation for FALS because the gene is located on an autosome – a chromosome that both males and females share. *Dominant* refers to the fact that a person only needs one gene to have the mutation that leads to a risk for ALS. Someone who has FALS would have one copy of the gene with a mutation and one copy of the gene without a mutation, giving that person's offspring a fifty percent chance of also inheriting the gene defect and getting ALS. That is the science and those are the odds, regardless of how the pattern may look on any given family tree.

The SOD1 discovery, based as it was on studies of familial ALS, also gave them pride. Their providing of first the details of pedigree, then of their actual DNA, which they believed lead to this discovery, made the families feel that they or their ancestors had made a significant contribution to science. It supported those in the family who were activists, giving them a sense of accomplishment and an argument against those who may have denied the hereditary nature of their form of the disease, or who—while not denying it—didn't want to get involved. Tennie's genealogical records were a contribution to an understanding that in some people ALS is inherited; now scientists were establishing that inheritance at the cellular level.

The SOD1 discovery also gave them a new way of contributing. One of Susan Lynaugh's roles as a family activist is to help recruit FALS families and patients to the cause. Family members can contribute by supplying the details of heredity to researchers such as Diane McKenna-Yasek, or their DNA in some form, or their bodies if they have been affected by the disease and will join a clinical trial, or their organs after death. She has spoken eloquently in meetings and webinars about how important it is that the FALS families sign up for the fight.

Shortly after 1993 family members also had the option of being tested themselves. It soon became possible to undergo testing to be entered into the FALS database as a carrier of the gene or not. It is also possible, of course, to find out whether you personally carry the defective gene. That decision – a very difficult one – will be discussed later.

Finally, the discovery of the SOD1 gene defect made possible, within a year, the creation of a mouse model. Today, mice have been genetically modified and have given birth to many other mice that have the SOD1 gene defect. These mice show signs of the disease within months of their birth, at first in one place, and then the disease progresses along lines very similar to its progression in humans – just a much shortened timetable. These murine subjects have become pervasive and invaluable to researchers. Models have also been created in fruit flies and rats, worms, even fish. Rats are enough larger than mice so that scientists can study spinal fluids or even test pumps to put fluids into their spinal cords.

· · · · ·

The Farrs of Northern Vermont—the Langmaids, Vances, Priors, Lynaughs, Longchamps, and Myricks actually acquired their pride and their hope later, as there were no activists in 1993. Five years later, a young man in the family—one of Tennie Toussaint's great-grandchildren—began to show symptoms of muscle weakness. That is when the Danville Farrs got back in touch with neurologists and ALS experts at Massachusetts General Hospital, and a new generation of activists within the family was born. Their involvement increased the awareness of all in the family, and they realized Grammy Tennie's contribution to an understanding of FALS, and the contribution of the farmer from Burke who, generations before, somehow made his way to Montreal to meet with the famous Dr. William Osler. They took pride in having been part of something and vowed to stay current and to find new ways to contribute to the science of a cure.

Palliative Care

Guides for patients with ALS use a variety of terms to describe what medical science can do for the patient with a definite diagnosis and progressing symptoms. Patients can "manage the disease." They can seek out a "comprehensive, interdisciplinary or multidisciplinary" clinic for their care. Such a clinic may include the attentions of a neurologist, physical therapist, occupational therapist, speech pathologist, dietitian, social worker, orthotist (a fitter of orthopedic appliances), pulmonologist, respiratory therapist, gastroenterologist, general surgeon, and psychologist or psychiatrist. ALS is not untreatable, the books say; it can be "managed aggressively," and "interventions can markedly enhance your quality of life."

Medicines may be prescribed to treat specific symptoms: hyoscyamine or scopolamine for drooling, inhalation breathing treatments with saline or acetylcysteine for thick phlegm, liquid lorazepam for the scary sensation of being unable to breathe called laryngospasm, various medicines for depression and for the uncontrollable laughter or crying (Pseudobulbar Affect), and there are a variety of options for cramping, spasms and pain. Patients may take oxybutynin or tolterodine tartrate for urinary urgency, over the counter stool softeners for constipation, and clonazepam or pramipexole for the periodic leg movements which can disturb sleep. Patient manuals also recommend a list of prescription medicines to treat fatigue and the symptoms that accompany it, such as insomnia, headache, irritability and anxiety.

In addition, patient manuals recommend physical therapy and various life changes for dealing with the symptoms of the disease, such as mild, tolerable exercises – carefully designed for help with flexibility or strength or aerobic capacity—in the early stages of the disease to stave off deconditioning and fatigue. ALS patients learn to eat differently, taking small bites, swallowing frequently, washing food down with sips of liquid, and tucking their chins down while swallowing. They learn to sleep in different positions or in different locations, such as in a recliner or hospital bed. Often, lying flat causes breathing difficulties. Patients may try satin sheets to help in repositioning themselves in the night.

Then, there are the machines. A patient's home may be littered with various apparatus that have been used or are being used to help him be comfortable, move about the house, or reposition himself from chair to bed to bath. A relatively young medical specialty is practiced by physiatrists, who practice the specialty of physical medicine and rehabilitation. Dr. Lisa Krivickas, in her chapter in *Amyotrophic Lateral Sclerosis: A Guide for Patients and Families* provided an overview of rehabilitation issues. "For the person with ALS," she writes, "this means rehabilitation to the optimal functional performance that is achievable given the stage of the disease." Krivickas acknowledged that all patients go through the stages of further debilitation. They need to order the equipment to be there when they'll need it. For example, for movement around the neighborhood, then the house, almost every patient will rely on a series of aids for balance and locomotion from a cane, to a walker, to a light wheel chair used only for outings, to a self-propelled chair with the big wheels, to a motorized chair.

Assistive technology is the term used for the practice of helping patients with communication, environmental control, seating and wheelchair movement, and worksite modification. New technology is being created every day to help patients manage the tasks of living at home with whatever capabilities they have, such as using voice commands to turn on the light, the wave of a hand or finger control to raise the shades, the eyes to type and browse the internet, or a puff of air from the lungs to control a wheelchair.

A special high-tech home in the Boston area—funded partly through donations from a current patient—contains infrared transmitters in the ceilings. The transmitters are connected to the home's master computer in the basement, which in turn can send the patient's signals to open and close doors, summon an elevator, turn up the heat, lower the shades, or turn down the lights.

For communication and for swallowing, patients may receive the services of a speech-language pathologist. Common difficulties are loss of speech clarity, loss of volume, hypernasal speech, slurring, choking, aspiration (the entrance of food or liquid into the lungs), or cognitive changes such as recalling words. A speech pathologist may help the patient with breath grouping – limiting the number of words per effort – to avoid losing breath and volume toward the end of a sentence. Here, technology in the form of a microphone may also help, and a home can be wired with speakers in several rooms. A sort of retainer can be fitted to the patient's mouth for modulating the nasal quality of speech.

Caregivers and the patient may also discuss strategies for communication to try to minimize the frustrations. As with stutterers and others with speech difficulties, ALS patients usually want to continue talking as long as they can and may actually be less touchy about the subject than their conversation partners. They want to be told if they are not understood rather than for their partner or a visitor to pretend to understand them. Krivickas suggests that speech partners give the patient feedback on what they understood and what they didn't ("I didn't get that last part after _____."). While they are still able to speak clearly, some patients do some voice banking; they may record a number of phrases or signature expressions, for storage in a computer for later use.

Once the ability to talk is lost, patients opt for some low-tech options, and then usually today go increasingly high-tech. In some patients, those with the bulbar form of the disease, voice may be lost before upper motor control. They may be able to point or to type for quite a while after losing the ability to produce intelligible speech. Two low-tech devices are simple letter and word boards used by pointing, or a transparent letter board, through which the patient and partner link eyes through a desired letter. Telecommunication devices for the deaf allow users to type their phone messages (if the receiver has such a device). Of course, for those with the dexterity, email and texting are options.

Today, most patients in their middle-to-late stages use keyboards on a screen which is placed directly in front of them. If the patient still can direct his head movements, a small reflective sticker on his head can be detected by a sensor on the computer to act as a mouse. Word-prediction and abbreviation-expansion features in word processing programs can complete a word which the patient begins. Electronic eye gaze systems enable a person to choose a letter simply by looking at it. The system is programmed to select the letter after the patient gazes on it for a predetermined time. Patients can type a phrase or full sentence, which then is converted to voice and is heard as a full phrase, not word-for-word. In very late stages, the patient can only blink, or signal Yes or No in some subtle way. Family and caregivers become adept at reading these subtle signals, and even the emotions behind them. They can read an emphatic Yes and an emphatic No.

The final, or at least next, frontier in speech technology is a brain-computer interface, in which a patient's thoughts are translated into actions. Electrodes implanted in the brain may one day enable a patient to focus on a letter or a message which is then spoken by a computer. The Brain Gate group of "transformative technologies" has as its motto "Thought into Action." The science is called a neural interfacing system. The system includes the electrode array implanted in the part of the brain which controls motor activity, one hundred gold wires which connect the array to a pedestal which extends through the scalp right on top of the head, an external cable which is simply plugged into the pedestal at the start of a session, and a set of computers that can store and analyze data. In addition, the firm's intellectual property includes software that will analyze the data and translate it into signals to control computer applications.

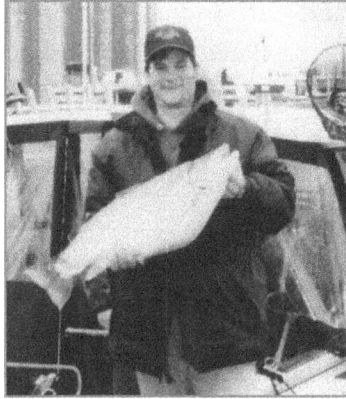

Curtis Vance, fishing,
Lake Ontario 1999.

CHAPTER 6

Curtis

In the summer of 1998, Curtis Vance was living a good life. A hard worker, he was employed as a logistics technician at IBM in Essex Junction three twelve-hour days per week, and worked on construction for Jon Webster Foundations back home in Danville two days per week. He was strong and fit, twenty-five years old.

He lived in New Haven, Vermont with his girlfriend Heidi Erdmann and their dog Wofosi. Heidi was working as an assistant tennis pro at the Basin Harbor Club in Vergennes. They had met in Danville, where Heidi's parents had a cottage on Joes Pond, when Heidi was only fifteen and Curtis seventeen. Heidi was a Connecticut girl from a wealthy suburb, Curtis very much a local boy from a family of many generations in northern Vermont. They had seen each other only during summers until she was twenty and going to college in Middlebury.

Curtis was the grandson of Clara Langmaid and great-grandson of Tennie Toussaint. He was one of five boys of Linda and Roy Vance. They were Christopher Roy, Craig Reginald, Curtis

Roger, Cary Ryan, and Carl Rodney. Within the family, according to his mother, Curtis may have had the label of "spoiled." That was because Curtis was the next child born to Roy and Linda after they had lost a baby boy, Charles, to crib death. Linda and Roy raised Curtis with that fear of losing him and may have been overprotective of him, she said.

Curtis had always been an active, physical guy. At Danville High School, he had been a member of the soccer, basketball, baseball and cross-country teams, as well as vice president of the student council. He had also been a popular kid and a caring friend. His mother Linda recalls that more than once the family took in other kids who were having troubles at home. Curtis and his brothers would bring them home like stray dogs and make room for them for a few months.

To his brother Craig, Curtis was known as "the worker." He was the guy to call if you needed something done around your house, because he was skilled and always willing to help. He was also known for his sense of humor. Actually, the whole family is. Active and popular in the small town, the boys were known for their good-natured fun. They all tended to be leaders. As Linda put it, "I wouldn't say that any of my kids sat in the second row." Curtis's high school graduation present was a red Ford Mustang.

After high school, not wanting to go to college, Curtis took a job with his father's company, which cleared brush and trees from under power lines. It was a second-generation business, started by his grandfather Lane. Curtis's father Roy kept pushing college, and he also insisted that Curtis keep looking for another job. Finally, after a back-breaking year on his father's crew, Curtis announced he would like to attend Vermont Technical College and enroll in its two-year building trades program, thereby satisfying both his parents' demand for further schooling and a degree and his own focus on learning practical skills. He attended VTC in Randolph, starting in the fall of 1991.

At VTC, he did well, graduating with honors. He also held leadership positions there, acting as a dorm proctor, but he was no angel. One of his tasks as a dorm proctor was to obtain liquor for his charges, which he transported in his own car, which by that time was a brown Cadillac. Curtis seems to have had the knack of quickly gaining the trust and friendship of people, such as liquor storeowners. The Caddy had actually been a gift from a stranger who had been helped by Curtis when the car broke down in Danville and who had then just given the disabled car to Curtis, who was under age at the time. His high school yearbook shows all of his friends piled into the Caddy. The impractical red Mustang and the Cadillac were gone by the end of college, to be replaced by a Ford pickup.

Graduating in 1993 with a degree in building trades from Vermont Tech, which prides itself on having a very high employment rate for its graduates, Curtis interviewed for jobs and was actually offered one in Hawaii, but he turned it down. He was a Vermont boy and a family guy. He took the job instead at IBM in Essex Junction, working three days per week. His relationship with Heidi deepened and after she graduated from Middlebury in 1997, they began to live together.

In August of 1998, Curtis felt that carrying a bunch of building materials up a flight of steps was more difficult than it should have been. He was generally tired, and his right bicep ached. He first questioned his own busy schedule, working twelve-hour shifts for IBM, then driving to Danville to work construction on other days. He wondered whether he had eaten something wrong. There had been some poorly cooked pork; maybe he had trichinosis. Curtis tried to get more rest, eat better and drink lots of water. He began to sleep twelve hours per night, but he still felt poorly at the start of the day and really lousy by the end of the day.

Something was wrong. What seems hard to understand is that neither Curtis nor his family thought at that stage that what was wrong was ALS. It had been twenty-five years, Curtis's whole lifetime, since Curtis's great-grandmother Tennie died, and the family wasn't at all sure that she had died of ALS. It had been thirty-six years since his grandmother Clara had died of something called progressive bulbar palsy, but in the meantime the family had put the disease out of their day-to-day thinking. As far as they knew, it had been generations since a male had died of the disease, and besides people typically acquired their first symptoms in their forties at the earliest; Curtis was male and only twenty-five. There were a lot of reasons to resist the terrible thought.

Linda's cousin Kelly Ralston had died of ALS in Georgia at age forty-three in 1988, but for some reason, that illness and death was not in the Vance family's calculations. In addition, Linda's aunt Rena Longchamps had died the same year in Burke Hollow, but Curtis's family was not aware (and are still not convinced), in her case, that the cause of her death was ALS.

Ironically, the medical profession knew this was coming, but the Vermont branch of the family had not been in contact with neurologists in Burlington, or Lebanon, New Hampshire (where Dartmouth Hitchcock Medical Center was now located) or Boston for quite a few years. In fact, Curtis himself had not seen any doctor since he was an infant. He didn't know what hit him.

Curtis first went to a walk-in clinic at Dartmouth Hitchcock Medical Center in Lebanon on October 1, 1998. He was taken there by Heidi and his father. His mother was in Ohio on a business trip, selling candles. Linda had been an OB-Gyn nurse for twenty years but had changed careers, partly to spend more time with her family and in her community. At the clinic Curtis was given a long series of tests evaluating his strength and reflexes and vital organs, and blood was drawn for lab tests.

Curtis actually made a series of visits to Dartmouth Hitchcock over the next few weeks. Trichinosis was investigated, and the doctors began to look at the motor neuron diseases. In retrospect, the family says, there were definite signs of ALS, especially the muscle weakness but also the tell-tale twitching of the muscles. Nevertheless, after weeks of testing at DHMC, Curtis was still not diagnosed with ALS.

Returning from Ohio and realizing for the first time the seriousness of her son's illness, and the frightening possibility of the family disease, Linda knew that Boston doctors were aware of the family history. She then insisted that they get in touch with the doctors there with whom her grandmother had corresponded. Tell them that this patient is a member of the Farr family, she said, and they will want to see him. And they did, eventually speaking with nurse Diane McKenna-Yasek of Mass General's neurology team, who filled them in on the family history. It was sinking in to Linda that she might lose her son, as she had her mother and her aunt, to this inexorable disease.

Curtis went to Massachusetts General Hospital in mid-November. There, he was examined by neurologists, who gave him another long series of tests, now conducted with their awareness that he was a member of the Farr family that had a long history with ALS. In fact, that was Curtis's confirmation that he had the family disease. He was also informed that the family history included the A4V point mutation which results in a very fast-progressing form of the disease. Curtis was given six to twelve months to live.

Linda Vance does not quickly show her emotions. She maintains a poker face, even when she is telling a joke, or a moving family story. This mother of six and the sibling of four was now faced with losing another son. "I went through a series of emotions," Linda recalls, "including anger, why me, why him. I tried to make deals with the Lord. 'Lord, let this be something else; let it happen to someone else.' "

Coincidentally, right after the diagnosis the Vance family took one of its three-generation trips, this time a cruise in the Caribbean. Along on the trip were Curtis and Heidi, Linda and Roy, Linda's sister Susan Lynaugh and her husband Dwayne, brothers Craig and Chris, and Chris's wife Pam and their children. As Linda recalls it, on the cruise Curtis' symptoms were not too advanced, and his diagnosis not fully accepted; as a result the family could enjoy themselves and for periods of time keep thoughts of the disease at bay. The trip was good therapy. Today, a snapshot on Linda and Roy's refrigerator captures the spirit of the vacation: Curtis, Susan, Linda, Roy, Chris's wife Pam and their son Derek, sit in a circle around the edge of a big hot tub, all smiling through the steam. Curtis used a cane on the trip but he got around with the others. Home movies show him playing shuffleboard, swimming, and dining with the family as they all tried to ignore the symptoms and the future.

Returning from the trip and resuming treatment, Curtis now entered into a new stage in his relationship with his doctors. For months there had been a search to find and confirm a diagnosis. For this next stage, Curtis's doctors invited him to be a test subject in several trials, and they helped manage his palliative care. They helped him anticipate what each next stage would be and helped him obtain the medicine and equipment to manage his life and condition. Heidi became his nurse.

In late December of that year, 1998, Curtis returned to Dartmouth Hitchcock Medical Center for examination and to be prescribed Rilutek, the one drug which by that time was approved for patients with ALS. Rilutek is the brand name for Riluzole, manufactured by Sanofi-Aventis. Rilutek has been shown in trials to extend the life of patients. In a coincidence in the history of this disease, the final trial of Rilutek, which led to its approval by the FDA, was conducted with outpatients from the Hopital de la Pitié-Salpêtriere in Paris, where amyotrophic lateral sclerosis had first been identified 120 years before.

Developed and tested, then approved in 1995, Rilutek works by blocking sodium channels that are associated with damaged neurons. This reduces the flow of calcium ions and thus indirectly prevents the build-up of glutamate. Glutamate is one of those substances in the brain that seems to be essential for nerve cells to communicate with one another; however, too much glutamate may contribute to the damage of the motor neurons. Rilutek, then, is a chemical that inhibits the overproduction of a good thing in people whose brains tend to overproduce that good thing. It is a delicate balancing act and in fact Rilutek does not do very much. It has been approved by the FDA simply because it does seem to prolong life for ALS patients. When most effective, it extends a patient's life span only several months. Rilutek is most effective, studies have shown, when it is taken early. It has no effect after eighteen months, which is why Curtis's doctors wanted to get him on it quickly; they knew that he had approximately one year to live. For Curtis to be given a prescription for anything gave the family some hope.

Heidi quit her job and undertook the full-time role as Curtis's caregiver. In February, she and Curtis moved from New Haven to Danville and into his aunt and uncle's new home. Mary and Hollis Prior had been building a pretty little colonial style home on a cul-de-sac. Danville is a hill town; that is, when you drive west on Route 2 from the Connecticut River valley through St. Johnsbury to Danville you are climbing most of the way. Around Danville's pretty green, and on the roads branching off along the ridge from the village, there are many homes with sometimes spectacular views of the Franconia Range in New Hampshire, Mount Lafayette, the ski trails on Cannon Mountain, and to the north Mount Washington and the Presidential Range.

The white cape-style home of Hollis and Mary Prior looks southeast with views of the nearby green hills and the distant mountains of New Hampshire. Both interested in history and old designs, according to Hollis, he and Mary had spent quite a bit of time and travel in finding just the right design for what they imagined to be a style from the late 1700s or early 1800s. They had sold their previous home a year before, and moved into an apartment while their new home was designed and built. In both the floor plan and the details, they wanted authenticity, which they achieved through choices such as the use of wide, softwood boards for the floor, square cut nails, a center chimney, and twelve-on-twelve windows.

The home was their own project and pride and joy, and in fact Curtis had been one of the carpenters who worked on it. Working with Jon Webster and Chris Zangla, and using his school-learned building trades skills, Curtis and the crew had first built the Priors a carriage shed garage, and then been hired to build the house.

The Priors were very pleased and of course anxious to move in to the house when Heidi called. She and Curtis had been living in a second floor apartment in New Haven, and getting up those stairs was getting difficult for Curtis. Plus, they wanted to be closer to Curtis's home, so she asked about their new house in Danville. "You can stay there as long as you want," Hollis responded, and so Curtis and Heidi moved in.

The home did not have a bedroom on the first floor. It did have a deck out back, and Heidi and Curtis bought a hot tub for the deck, thinking it would be good therapy for Curtis's tight, painful muscles. This was endorsed by MGH doctors. In fact, Dr. Merit Cudkowicz, a relatively new member of MGH's ALS neurology team, remembers writing her first ever prescription for a hot tub. Later, a local welder, Gordon Hastings, made them a bracket to accept the Hoyer lift to help Curtis get in and out of the hot tub. Eventually, they added a roof over the deck. A bed was set up for Curtis in the living room.

While the Vance family began to accept the science that told them that their family had the inherited form of the disease, they continued to believe that its onset nevertheless needed a trigger. The inexorable nature of the disease, and the lack of virtually any progress in the treatment of the disease in the 130 years since it was identified, said to the Vances and Heidi that it was a mystery, and mysteries can be solved. They were not about to sit around and wait for the latest cure, or to consider only the offerings of medical science.

For his part, as the diagnosis set in and the symptoms mounted but were not yet debilitating, Curtis found a kind of peace, and began to notice and appreciate things as he was freed from the demands of work and home. He read more, he meditated, he looked at the mountains, and he talked to Heidi. He said that, although he knew his time was short, in another way he had been given time, a kind of blessed time that he may never have found in a busy life, or if he had died suddenly. "We've got these beautiful mountains," he explained as an example. "I've lived here my whole life and I saw them, but I never really noticed them and their beauty. Now I do all the time."

Curtis continued to make monthly visits to Mass General. MGH and its doctors had taken over his care but also would ask him to be part of various clinical trials. As a member of the Farr family, Curtis felt that he was important to the neurologists there. In January of 1999, he was enrolled in a randomized, double-blind, placebo-controlled research trial of r-metHuBDNF, abbreviated and referred to as BDNF, standing for Brain Derived Neurotropic Factor. Manufactured by Amgen, BDNF was a synthetic protein similar to a protein naturally found in the nervous system. The hope was that this synthetic protein would perform the function that its natural form performed in enhancing the survival and function of damaged motor neurons. BDNF had already been studied by injecting it into the skin of over 1,400 patients without positive results. However, Dr. Cudkowicz and her team wanted to see if it would be more effective if injected directly into the spinal fluid, a process known as intrathecal injection. This would be accomplished by implanting an intrathecal pump into the patient's abdomen.

As in all double-blind studies, subjects of this study received one of two levels of dosage through the pump, or a placebo solution of saline. Neither the patient nor his doctor would know which group Curtis was in. (In fact, he was in the low-dose group, which his family would learn two years later.) The effectiveness of the solution would be measured by broad measurements of Curtis's continued muscle function. The study was also a test of the delivery system, the SynchroMed Infusion System, manufactured by Medtronics, which was still investigational, although it had been in use for eleven years. MGH was enrolling eighteen study participants of 270 anticipated in the US, Europe and Canada. The study was being funded by the pharmaceutical companies Amgen and Medtronics.

Consent forms for patients in a clinical trial list the science behind the therapy, and possible side effects, but they also list the possible benefits. The trial offered the hope that, if the medicine was effective, it could be continued. The pump was implanted, and Curtis went home to await the results. The surgery immobilized Curtis for several weeks and resulted in severe headaches.

Curtis and Heidi, with support from family and friends, settled into a life devoted to the search for some comfort and relief for Curtis. While remaining open to the latest possible treatments from medical science, its drug trials and therapeutic inventions, Heidi and Curtis also set out to harness what they referred to as "the healing powers of community." Beginning in April, they started holding weekly healing circles in their home. Neighbors, family, and friends came to sit with Curtis and by whatever means, extend to him their healing energy. They brought refreshments – a bread, a plate of brownies – and circling around him as he lay in his recliner, they did breathing exercises, or lay hands on him, or told old positive stories of the past, directing positive energy to the stricken man. Facilitated by neighbor and family friend Diana Webster, Jon Webster's wife, the sessions lasted one hour. They were usually held on Thursday nights. Depending on the weather, they were held in their home, or outdoors, and sometimes at a local restaurant. For the first healing circle held in April, twelve people attended, but the numbers grew. The family estimates that the weekly gatherings may have averaged forty people. One week there were 150 people.

As Linda put it, "In the Bible it says that where there are two or more people gathered in His name, then there will be healing." Facilitator Diana Webster compared it to the healing energy of prayer, "just in a different context." Neighbor Jenness Ide was quoted in a newspaper article about the circle as saying, "The disease makes me feel powerless, absolutely powerless. This is one way of getting some power."

The theory behind the healing circles was from the ideas of Dr. Wayne London, what Dr. London calls the metaphysical approach to disease. Just as a certain Type A personality is associated with heart disease, London argued in a 2007 essay, so are certain personality traits and environmental factors associated with ALS. "Group warrior memories," London called them, noting that ALS appears more frequently in certain professions – soldiers, athletes, nurses, police and fire people – than in the general population. Their activities as well as the "warrior place" in which they grew up may trigger the disease. This is another way of explaining clusters of ALS cases.

As has been discussed earlier, geographical clusters of ALS patients have been of interest to doctors as much as the familial clusters. Researchers reason that a cluster of patients opens up an area of study to figure out what aspect of the environment is causing the disease to appear at a much larger rate than usual. Herbicides, pesticides, fertilizers, heavy metals, and diet have been studied as potential causes or triggers in these places, and London suggested that "one unknown environmental factor is not physical but metaphysical, such as the memory of a group or individual experience."

"This metaphysical approach," London wrote in 2007, "suggests an immediate, cost effective and preventative healing strategy—non-attachment to prior group warrior experiences." Basing his theories on the practice of indigenous people in Australia and elsewhere, London proposed a group healing practice in which the group helps the patient, and his partner, to detach themselves from the "prior warrior experience."

The stages of ALS, in addition to being characterized by symptoms, are characterized by attitudes, those of the patient and those of his old circle of friends and acquaintances. People don't know what to do when they hear of the dire diagnosis. Some stay away, not because they are weak friends or distant family to begin with, but because they don't want to see their friend or relative in such a state, or because they can't handle the pain. Patients see their circle get smaller. One ALS patient suggested that it is also because people are too busy and—especially once the patient is confined to his or her home—it requires more time and effort to see an old friend. This man used to meet regularly for coffee and conversation, and much political arguing, with a group of men at the local diner. There came a point however, when it was harder for him to get to the diner, and he felt uncomfortable there due to his difficulty talking. He stayed at home, where a few of the men visited him. Many ALS patients see that circle shrink to a very small one, comprised perhaps of a pastor, a single friend, and close family.

Not so with Curtis. He seemed to enjoy company, as Linda described it, and instantly made people feel at home. A visit to Curtis was not that grim. "He didn't act that depressed or sad even," Linda said. "He knew where he was going. He would wink and smile when that was all he could do."

Participation in the healing circles indicated a belief in miracles. "I don't think we have any other choice," said Linda, his mother. Because there was the family history, and the big family to follow, she explained, "If this doesn't turn around, it gives no hope for anybody else in the family." Any miracle – medical or spiritual – that could save Curtis could promise hope for the rest of the family. The Methodist minister, Carol Borland, was a regular visitor. Other neighbors and friends came by for particular purposes: to read to Curtis, to massage his muscles, to watch sports on TV. "There was a kind of hope," Linda said, "but not necessarily for Curtis to live."

Curtis began to have difficulty breathing in April. This symptom is troubling. It shows a deterioration in the bulbar muscles which has consequences for talking, eating, and for breathing comfortably enough to allow sleeping.

The family took a trip to Holmes County in Ohio in April, to visit an Amish family that the Vances knew through their mutual interest in Belgian draft horses. It was a pleasant trip, as Linda remembers, as the two large families celebrated Easter together. Curtis enjoyed the blossoming of spring. He marveled at the number of cardinals, the red bird being rare in New England. Curtis indulged his love for Coblenz chocolates. He and Heidi bought two hickory-branch rockers.

In May, Curtis returned to Mass General for five days for a battery of tests and to be fitted for a BiPAP machine for help with breathing. BiPAP stands for Biphasic Positive Airway Pressure. It is a form of non-invasive help with breathing, non-invasive meaning that there is no surgical insertion. The machine is simply a mask that helps the patient breath by forcing air into his lungs through both the nostrils and mouth at just a little above ambient pressure. The pressured air helps with both breathing in (inspiration) and breathing out (expiration). The mask is attached by tubes to a pump which filters and gently pushes room air into the tight-fitting mask. Bi-level refers to the fact that with this machine, the inspirational air is a little higher in pressure than the expirational air.

That summer, Heidi's sister Tricia came to live with them and to help care for Curtis. Curtis, Heidi and Tricia often spent time outdoors. A cement pad had been poured for Curtis's chair and for the hickory rockers. Curtis enjoyed sitting out there, watching Mary and Hollis plant the gardens and trees in their new yard, and looking at the mountains.

Curtis was also able to pursue his interest in NASCAR stock car racing, especially in the fortunes of his favorite driver, Tony Stewart, the driver of Number 14 (much to the annoyance of his brother Craig, a fan of Number 24 Jeff Gordon). A Danville friend, Dorothy "Petey" Blackadar, who with her now-deceased husband Archie had long been involved with NASCAR, contacted Stewart, told him of Curtis's condition and his interest, and put Stewart in touch with Curtis. Curtis even got to visit pit row when the Winston Cup circuit came to New Hampshire Motor Speedway in Loudon in July.

Also that summer, due to the kindness of friends, Curtis took a memorable fishing trip to Lake Ontario. Heidi and Curtis and two fishing buddies, John Coffin and Vinnie Cartularo, spent several days fishing for king salmon near Pulaski, New York, a salmon mecca. Curtis was in a wheelchair by the time of this trip. A photo of Curtis proudly displaying his own trophy catch, next to the mounted salmon, adorns the wall of his father's barber shop in the basement of their house.

Before Curtis's illness, Heidi and Curtis had planned to get married someday. That was definite. After his symptoms and diagnosis, however, Curtis was reluctant. He didn't want to marry Heidi and then die shortly after, he said. By October, however, he had changed his mind. There were a number of reasons. The wedding would sanctify their marriage before God. It would seal their commitment to each other. It would make Heidi his guardian and his legal care supervisor before death and his legal heir after death. Curtis suggested that the wedding be held in the spring when everything was in bloom. They thought that Curtis had many months to live. But that fall, because Curtis's health was so fragile, they decided to hold the wedding as soon as possible.

The wedding took place on November 27, 1999 at North Congregational Church in St. Johnsbury before five hundred guests. Curtis was in a wheelchair, his four brothers standing as groomsmen, waiting for Heidi as she came down the aisle with her father. Heidi wore her aunt's wedding dress. Dressed in a dark suit but with his BiPAP mask shielding both his face and his emotions, Curtis smiled as broadly as he could, and showed his delight in his eyes.

Curtis was growing very weak as December began. He was also anxious, having difficulty breathing and sleeping. The BiPap just wasn't keeping up. He was also having difficulty knowing whether it was time for him to go, to accept the moment of the end. Sensing that Curtis needed some sort of release, Heidi told Linda that Linda was the one who needed to give him that release. Curtis didn't want to die because he was afraid of letting his mother down: that's the way Linda remembers Heidi's message. Linda knew that she had to give Curtis her blessing. She also knew that she just couldn't do it in person, extemporaneously, to "just run to him and hold him and tell him that it was all right," because she would just break down and not get it out. She decided that she would write him a letter, and that she would then read it to him.

On December 18, the plan was to take Curtis to the family's hunting camp—The Stagger Inn they called it—in North Danville. Family and friends would hold a Christmas party there. It was well planned. The road to the camp was lighted with luminaria. A hay wagon took the partiers to the camp. Someone had welded an angel, which hung over the camp.

Linda wrote her letter that afternoon and read it to Curtis

before he went to the party. "I knew in that moment that it was up to me who gave birth to him twenty-six years ago to now give him the freedom that he needed to die in peace," Linda would recall, and so with Roy and Heidi present, she sat with Curtis and read him the letter, all 2000 words. It was actually a history of Linda's journey as a survivor in this family decimated by ALS, and the set of beliefs she had come to embrace about the meaning of those losses to a Christian woman who believed in God's love. That reading went well, she thought. Curtis loved it. Then he went to the party.

The next day, December 19, everyone sensed that the end was near. Heidi called Linda and Roy and told them to come. Word got around and in fact between thirty and forty people gathered in that small living room around Curtis's bed, as he lay struggling with his breathing. Heidi was at his side. His niece and nephew sat on the bed. Linda sat on the end of the bed, her back to her dying son, and read her letter again:

> *Dear Curtis,*
>
> *This is a love letter from my heart to yours. I could not tell you in person what I wanted to say or how I feel because I would only cry and so I am using the only way that I know to tell you what is deep within my soul about things. I love you from the very depths of my being, and you are a favorite son among a group of six favorites.*
>
> *Where shall I begin? Perhaps from the very beginning is a good place. When my mother died of this disease I was a student at nursing school and knew that my mother was sick, but I did not know that she was going to die so I did not ever say goodbye or that it was okay or that I would be okay, and I missed that.*

We were not a huggy-kissy family and so I do not remember that part of my mom nor was I ever brought up to do that, so your illness has been hard for me in that respect, but you and your healing circle have helped me 100% or maybe 99% to come to terms with my grief and love for her and for you, too.

When my aunt came down with the disease she called me aside and told me never to have children because I would not want them to get this disease through me now would I? However, I decided that there are a lot of diseases and things that can happen to people so I would go ahead and have my family as I had planned, and if anyone would get this I was sure it would only be me anyway, and I could handle it for myself.

Little did I dream that one of my babies would have it, but I have to tell you that I don't regret for even one moment that I had each and every one of the six of you, disease or no disease, because I love each of you more than life itself. If it would possibly change anything at all I would gladly die for you today and not be afraid to do that, but God does not give me that choice. So my mother and my aunt died unafraid and ready to live in a much more wonder-ful place as will you and I and all of us someday, and I honestly believe that.

Curtis, please trust me that you will be happy and free and with people who love you as much as I do, and your father and your brothers and your wife Heidi and all your many friends and relatives both born and unborn will be with you in a moment because I believe that time in Heaven is measured in moments. I have never knowingly told you a lie, and

I know from God's word and from his whispers to me that this is true because would a God who made the sun and the moon and the stars and the rainbow as a promise give us less than perfect in Heaven?

When your brother Charles died I was not prepared, and he was so very little I could only wonder about God's wisdom in taking him from me, but I have always secretly thought that my mother needed him more at the moment than I did, and God knew that I would have you and your brothers so he chose him for her. I have always felt sad for myself in his parting but kind of happy for her because she was truly a great and wonderful mother whose arms were empty, and God knew that I would understand.

When I became pregnant with you, I was so very happy that I would do anything to protect you and so I quit smoking, ate only the best foods and gave birth to you in a 20 minute rush into the world. You were always so active and so beautiful and so in a hurry to get things done right that I have wondered at your ability and your love of people and the land and life. When I was still in the hospital with you I learned about angels from my mother because one night I awoke to find her sitting on the end of the bed, and she looked just like an angel with my mother's face, and she told me not to worry or fear because she would and was taking care of my baby. I did not know at the time that she meant you too. But trust me again Curt when I tell you that she will love you as much as I have loved you, and you will recognize her as being good and kind and loving as you are too.

When my dad died a few years ago I wasn't ready for that either, but I knew that he would be happier *with my mom, and it was starting to get harder for him to get around with his asthma and his hip pain, and I felt maybe it was a blessing that he did not have to suffer. He was such a great man, a lover of people and his family and a real farmer, a man who took real good care of God's land. He had time in his occupation to really see the world for what it really is and to appreciate God's love for us and his plan.*

Maybe by now God has him tending his apple orchards in Heaven, and perhaps you can help him as he always had to have another Fronzo in the village to teach and train so I will think of you when you go to join him working with him in the orchard. In the future whenever I see an apple tree in bloom or laden with fruit I will think of the two of you together, and I will love you both with all my heart.

Next to die was my very best friend Nancy, whom I loved so much and cared about and did fun things with. She was a true friend who tried to keep me straight, hard as that is. She was so very very sick that I could not wish her to live on this earth like that. But it was then that I really started talking to God to try to get him to perform some kind of a miracle to "save her" for my own selfish reasons. The thing that I didn't realize at the time was that God was prepared to offer her much more in Heaven.

When she died I was in Ohio, and I screamed and cried and yelled at God WHY WHY WHY? And when he answered it was with love and peace and he said to me, Linda I am prepared to offer her peace and love with no more pain or sorrow so be happy for her. I am. He also told me to go out into the world and become a friend to all men, which I have tried and will try even harder to do.

Grandpa Vance was the next to die, and you pretty much know all of that. I did love him as we all did, and he left us with a great feeling of peace. I think he was a little frustrated because his body did not want to do what his mind wanted it to, and I would be grumpy then too.

And now there is you Curtis, and you will always be my baby, and I will never want to let you go which is very selfish on my part I know, and it is okay to die and to leave this earth for a much better place, but it is really not easy for me to say that. I know why God wants you to come and be with him because you are a very special person.

I know now that I will forget to tell you some of the things that I think and feel in the letter, but I will make little P.S.›s to you for the rest of my life, so when you are up there tending those apple trees and sowing seeds of friendship and helpfulness every-where, whenever you hear P.S.›s listen up because it will be your mother talking to you or perhaps your father because he has a lot he wants to say to you, too, and just doesn›t know how. He cries every day and cares more for you than his life too. You know him, and he would do anything in his power to make you well. Every day he prays to God for a miracle and just cannot believe that it hasn›t happened yet. Today he said through his tears that he didn›t understand because he had prayed and begged God, and God hadn›t done a thing. What is wrong? Well Curtis, perhaps God has performed a miracle.

Your very life is a miracle; the love of your family to you and you to them is a miracle; your wife and lover of your soul and you of hers is a miracle; your relationship with the community and your love for them and they for you is a miracle; the healing circle is a miracle and how it has changed all our lives for the better; the love of your dog and you for him is a miracle; all of the events of the last year have been small miracles snowballing into one large one; the miracle of a new family for you with sisters and in-laws who love you with all their hearts; the miracle of the Wedding of the Century and everyone who was there will never forget the love they shared with the two of you, and those who were not there have heard what they missed and also want to share in the love.

I guess to sum up the miracle at this time of year, it is the story of Jesus' birth, and the idea that because of your illness the whole community looks at life and this season a little differently as is shown in the heart and soul of a little eight year old boy who didn't want Santa to bring him anything this year, only health for a man he barely knew. I guess you could say, that was the reward and miracle you should receive, blind faith and trust in a Santa or in God who can do anything. Daddy and I remember another little boy who at the age of 14 also didn't want anything big for Christmas, just new basketball uniforms for his team, so that they could be proud to compete.

Yes Curtis, you have taught us a lifetime of things in these few short years, the miracle of love, how to work hard and love our neighbors. You were never judgmental or boastful. You have loved the land and the world, and the animals. You have always been a good boy and now, an even greater man that we are proud to call son, brother, relative and friend. Oh, how we have all loved you Curtis in our own special way.

And yes Curt, your father and I and your family and all your friends will continue to cry for you because we love you so very much and because it is not easy for us to let go or give up. I guess my house and cellar attest to that for me, but when it is your time we will let you go, because in the end it is your reward and what is best for you. Know wherever you are, or we are, or whatever you are doing, or we are doing, we will all, your Dad, Me, Chris, Pam, Craig, Cary, Carl, Alysia, Derek, all your relatives, and all your new relatives, all your friends and people who barely know you will always love you very much, you Curtis are our Angel forever.

Love,

Mom

As Linda read the letter, her son died. As she finished it, all present acknowledged that he had stopped breathing as he heard her words. Heidi took off the BiPAP mask, she and others kissed Curtis. People gradually filed out.

The funeral service for Curtis was held at the large North Congregational Church in St. Johnsbury on December 23. Rev. Rona Tyndall of the Danville Congregational Church conducted the service.

Shortly after Curtis's death, his mother and his aunts conceived plans for a memorial orchard and a foundation to raise money for ALS research. The Curtis Vance Memorial Orchard was born. The family chose a lovely spot on family land near Grandma Tennie's sugarhouse on a hillside with a view to the southeast, a spot that had been one of Curtis's favorites. The idea was to create a quiet, beautiful spot for people to visit, and to use the space to hold several fundraising events per year. "We wanted a serene natural setting as a memorial to Curtis, who loved the outdoors," said his Aunt Susan.

In the spring following Curtis's death, there was a gathering to plant the orchard. Contributors paid one hundred dollars each for a chance to plant an apple tree in memory of their loved ones. Local artist Joe Hallowell donated a welded "iron tree," which was placed in a fieldstone foundation with a cornerstone selected from Grandma Tennie's sugarhouse. The site would serve as a quiet refuge open to the public, as well as the site of the family's annual fundraising picnic and auction.

That event is held every June and draws people from the community, the area, and beyond. The family serves a large delicious buffet meal with a barbecue, and holds an auction of donated items. Curtis's brother Craig serves as auctioneer.

Curtis's uncle Clif's contribution to the event has been to build, over the years, a large log lodge with balconies, a wrap-around porch, and dormers overlooking the orchard, a small pond, Clif's hay fields, and the distant view. The lodge is surrounded by beautiful fieldstone terraces, walls and stairs created by Phil Beattie. The family plans to offer The Apple Log Lodge as a function space for events, and a bed-and-breakfast. "We wanted to create a long-lasting, physical place," explained his aunt Susan, "not just another website and a charitable foundation."

The Curtis Vance Memorial Orchard has also sponsored a small market in North Danville village. The little one-room space, called "the pie shack" by the family, offered fresh-baked pies and pastries, jams and jellies, and other homemade, preserved foods from the early spring into the fall each year. Operated on an honor system, the market had a cooler of cold drinks, and even hot coffee. Linda and Susan's creations, such as tongue pickles, Thanksgiving relish, dilly beans in a jar, apple butter and maple peanut butter may also be purchased by mail-order via the Orchard's website, and are sold at area festivals and events, and at the nearby Great Corn Maze.

Since the creation of the orchard and the fundraising

operation, the family has donated $10,000 – $15,000 per year to the search for a cure for ALS. The bulk of the contributions have gone to Massachusetts General Hospital and the work of Dr. Merit Cudkowicz and her team at the Northeast ALS Consortium. Dr. Cudkowicz has visited the orchard.

The orchard has become a refuge and even a destination. A guestbook is kept on the site, and in it visitors—some from out of the state—have recorded their impressions and their appreciation for the facility. A common entry: "What a beautiful, peaceful place, and what a lovely tribute."

The very public illness and death of Curtis Vance brought the Farr family disease to the attention of the extended family and the community. After Curtis, there was no way to honor Grammy Tennie's apparent wish to hide the facts, to let the family live their lives in Danville without this cloud hanging over them. Curtis's illness was a wakeup call. It made activists of Linda and Susan, and it educated the whole family.

Sadly, it would not be long before ALS again came to Danville. After Heidi moved out, Hollis and Mary Prior moved into their precious new home in 2000. They were both working at that time but retired in 2007. Having reached retirement at age sixty-one in 2007, Mary said to Hollis that it looked like she had passed the age at which ALS usually strikes, but the disease, which had proven unpredictable in the family's past, would strike again, to two members of the family at once.

PART IV

ALS Today
(2000 – 2015)

Crisis and the End of Life Decision

More than half of all ALS patients die at home, and for a certain percentage of patients death follows a clear decision to let go. ALS patients at the end of life benefit from the services and the science of the hospice movement. A lot has been learned and shared about the events and the stages of the end of life, and patients and their families often turn to trained hospice caregivers to help make the last days precious rather than terrifying, a series of family events rather than an isolated and lonely life. Some guides for patients do not treat end-of-life issues but those that do recommend the hospice approach.

A relatively new movement, the hospice program is now Medicare certified. To receive hospice care under Medicare, the patient must have a physician-certified prognosis of less than six months to live. Hospice services may include physician services, nursing services with twenty four-hour call availability, social work services, a chaplain, and volunteers.

This final period in a patient's life can be a time for the family and close friends to gather, much to the relief and comfort of the patient, but that is often hard for family members. According to the writers of the hospice care chapter in the third edition of *A Guide for Patients and Families*, "doubt and distrust can derail a meeting before it has begun." The reason is that old wounds related to past favoritism, slightings, allegiances, feuds, and even previous mournings may emerge. Some family members may want to reopen those old wounds, on the one hand, or not want to attend a meeting, on the other hand. Some family members have legitimate opinions that talking only makes matters worse. In families with familial ALS that is even more likely to be the case, as different family members have developed different ways of coping with the "family curse," some denying it, some just not wanting to get into it, while others are devoting their lives to the study of and cure for the disease. Troubled families may need a skilled facilitator either from within the family or outside it.

For other families, however, the disease has brought the family together over the months, and they want to be together in these last days. Sometimes three or four generations gather. The ALS hospice guide suggests that the family relive the history of the disease, that they unburden themselves of guilt or fears that have been harbored, and that they talk about each other. It is a time to retell old family stories. The patient may be invited to share his or her current fears. Experts or family members with experience can then explain that death from ALS is usually quite peaceful and painless.

Families in these last stages may face difficult ethical and legal issues. The most common ethical dilemma is when or if to turn off a ventilator or other less-invasive breathing aid. If a patient does not wish to prolong his or her life by going on a ventilator, that is his or her right, and if it is clearly expressed then the family has an obligation to honor that wish. There may be conflict over that within the family, as loved ones plead with the patient and siblings to prolong life. The process of saying good-bye, of tying up loose ends, and getting one's affairs—financial and emotional—in order, takes time. Some family members might agree with the decision and may not be in denial that the end is near, but may still wish for more time.

Once a patient is on a ventilator, however, the decision to turn it off is very difficult. When first hitched up to a machine that breathes for him, a patient may still have his communication faculties and with patience can type out his carefully formed thoughts. After weeks, months, or even years on a ventilator, however, the

ALS patient's ability to communicate his intention may be severely limited. A certain movement up and down of the eyeballs may be his way of saying Yes. In Japan, it is against the law to turn off a ventilator once a patient is put on it. In the United States, however, a series of cases, including two ALS cases, has confirmed the patient's right of autonomy, and therefore his or her right to clearly signal a desire to be removed from a ventilator. In a third ALS case the court affirmed a woman's right to have her feeding tube removed against the wishes of her Roman Catholic hospital.

ALS patients rarely die alone. In most cases, the family and friends understand that the end is near and gather in a vigil. The cause of death is usually respiratory failure, as loved ones monitor the labored breathing until the end.
Obituaries often read that the patient died "surrounded by family and friends."

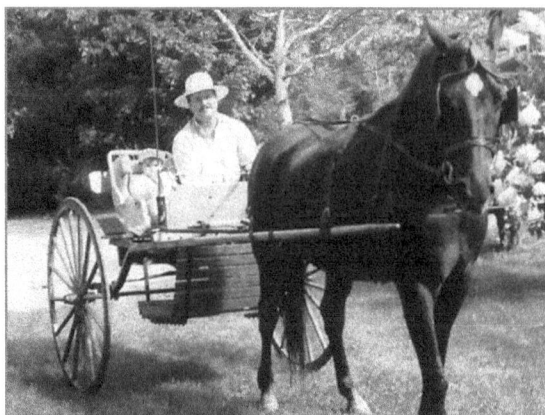

*Dennis Myrick, holding the reins,
with daughter Maura 1995.*

CHAPTER 7

Mary and Dennis

In 2009 cousins Mary Prior and Dennis Myrick lived in neighboring towns, Mary in Danville, Dennis in St. Johnsbury, Vermont. Both had grown up in or near North Danville village. They were twelve years apart, however, and had not been close cousins or playmates. When ALS first visited North Danville in 1962, Mary was sixteen years old, Dennis four. Mary was the daughter of Clara McGill and Forrest Langmaid, Dennis the son of Calista McGill and Charlie Myrick. They both grew up with some knowledge of FALS in the family. Mary had lost her mother Clara, her aunt Williamina, and her nephew Curtis. Dennis knew of ALS in his aunts, and in Curtis. Their grandmother Tennie in 1973, and their aunt Rena in 1988, may also have died of ALS, but their deaths were not uniformly attributed to ALS within the Vermont family.

ALS had left the Vermont branch of the family alone for twenty-six years, or so the family thought, but down in Georgia, they had heard, their cousin Kelton Ralston had died of ALS in

1988. In fact, Dennis was living and working in Georgia at the time. Then Curtis got sick in 1998, and Kelton Ralston's brother Kenneth died of ALS in Georgia in 2001. Mary and Dennis, then, knew the genealogical facts and the symptoms. They were sixty-three and fifty-one respectively in 2009, when they both began to notice muscle weakness. Mary had just retired from her career as a librarian; Dennis was a commercial property owner, businessman, and business consultant.

Mary was the second of five children. Early on she had acquired the nickname White Top due to her very light blonde hair. She had grown up in North Danville village, the daughter of a farmer. She graduated from Danville High School in 1964.

Mary and Hollis Prior met in 1967 when she was his secretary on her summer job in the office of the Vermont Department of Forest and Parks, where he was a pest control officer. She was twenty-one at the time and between her junior and senior years at the University of Vermont. Hollis was twenty-eight. They started dating and were married shortly after her graduation in 1968.

Hollis told me that Mary had been open about the family disease. In fact, he remembers being taken aside one day by Grammy Tennie. He was splitting wood for her at her home and she asked him to stop for a cup of tea. "She told me exactly what might happen," he recalls. That did not change his love for Mary, however, or their plans to have children. "It [ALS] really didn't play a big part in any of our decisions," Hollis said. He remembers the day, perhaps when Mary had turned 60, that she said to him, "I think we've passed it," referring to the usual age of onset of ALS.

Hollis worked for the Department of Forest and Parks for forty-three years, becoming an expert on pests and diseases that threaten Vermont's forests. He also became an expert on fruit tree diseases and pests. Mary's career had been as a librarian in several settings, most recently at the Barnet School. Along the way, Mary had earned her master's degree in library science from UVM. She had also worked at Danville's Pope Memorial Library and for the state library, and had trained herself to implement the use of computer technology as it arrived in schools and libraries in the nineties.

Mary and Hollis Prior had three children and two grandchildren. Both retired, they were active in their community. Mary was President of the Danville Historical Society, and a member of the Danville Women's Club. She played the organ and sang in the choir at the Danville Methodist Church. She was an outspoken Democrat. Hollis was active in the Historical Society too, and was known as the community's best informed arborist and fruit grower. In the area, he was the guy to call about an infestation in your apple trees, or for help planting an orchard, or bringing an old orchard back into production. As he explained it to me, "In retirement I was doing the same kind of work I did for my job, only I wasn't getting paid for it." He had designed and planted the orchard at the Curtis Vance Memorial Orchard site. For their devotion to community, Mary and Hollis were named Citizens of the Year in 1999. "The guardian angels of the town," they were called.

Dennis grew up in North Danville, in the village as a child, then on the North Danville Road between St. Johnsbury and the village. He too was the second child. He had an older brother, two younger brothers, and a younger sister. After graduating from Danville High School in 1975, he studied at a polytechnic university in Georgia and then worked in the printing trade there. He met his wife Dorene in North Danville, where her grandparents lived. They were married in 1981 and had three daughters in the first four years of their marriage, but it was a short, bitter marriage leading to divorce in 1992. Dennis and Dorene had moved back to Vermont, where Dennis continued in printing before getting involved in state government and politics. He ran several campaigns for office seekers and was an aide to State Senator John Carroll in the 1990s. Dennis was a Republican.

During that time, he studied at Woodbury College to become a paralegal, and eventually worked for attorney Deborah Bucknam in St. Johnsbury. He was employed as a general manager by Mathew Burak, a furniture parts maker. He held that job for seven years before deciding at age forty-five to go back to college. He enrolled at Lyndon State College and graduated in 2003 with a bachelor of science degree in business administration. He was then accepted into Vermont Law School, which he attended from 2003-2006. His learning during those years also included study trips to Russia, Finland, Italy and Spain. In addition to his law degree, he also earned a master's degree in environmental law at VLS.

Everyone I interviewed about Dennis for this book used similar terms to describe him. They all described him as very capable and likeable. According to Bernier Mayo, he was a "Renaissance Man," brilliant in several areas, including training and caring for horses, photography, painting and business. But they also described him as lacking in confidence, restless, and insecure about things such as his lack of formal education and his fitness and appearance. It was characteristic of Dennis to walk away from a success to go in search of something better, then to pour himself into the new thing and succeed at it, only to move on to something else. "He was always searching for the next opportunity," said Dave Redmond, who succeeded Dennis at Burak Furniture and knew him as a runner, business man and in Republican Party circles.

In recent years, Dennis had seen little of his daughters, now grown women in their twenties. In 1993, he remarried. He and his new wife Rosaleen had a daughter, Maureen, who was fifteen years old in 2009.

After graduating from law school, Dennis studied for the Vermont Bar Exam but never passed the full exam, a source of deep disappointment to him because he had a strong interest in the law and had hoped to be a practicing attorney. He had devoted himself to the study of law only to fail the exam by a very small margin. With his background in law and business, however, in 2006 Dennis set himself up as a consultant.

Myrick Management Inc. had offices on Eastern Avenue in St. Johnsbury. Among his clients were the Vermont Milk Company, Northend Hardwoods, and the Caledonia Kiln. The Vermont Milk Company was founded as a for-profit venture to provide Vermont farmers with a stable, high price for their milk. In a dairy production facility in Hardwick, the company had started by producing cheese and yogurt with milk from only five farms, and had idealistic goals of providing a fair, steady price for Vermont farmers' milk and growing a Vermont brand name. But higher milk and gasoline prices had put the company in arrears. Farmers weren't getting paid, plant workers were laid off. Dennis had been hired to try to rescue the company in 2008.

I first met Dennis in the fall of 2008 when he applied for help from the local Habitat for Humanity affiliate, for which I was a volunteer. The Myricks asked us to construct a ramp for his mother so that she could move into Dennis's home in St. Johnsbury. Calista had been injured in a car accident in April of 2005, and had been in several hospitals and rehabilitation centers. Dennis had ordered the materials to build the ramp but could not afford to hire professional carpenters to put it together. We at Northeast Kingdom Habitat for Humanity, just starting to organize an affiliate, did not have a very formal application process with income guidelines at the time, and Dennis said he would be paying the costs, so we sent a crew to his house for a one-day job. Dennis helped. I later learned from Dennis that another reason that he had asked for help was that he was feeling unusual fatigue and weakness in his daily activities. It was the kind of job that he, maybe with his dad Charlie, would have tackled on their own in the past, but Dennis did not feel up to it.

At this stage in his life and his career, Dennis was property rich but cash poor. He owned houses in Danville and St. Johnsbury, a hunting camp in Wheelock, and a business block in St. Johnsbury with a retail business, The Downtown Market and Creamery. He and Ro also owned Rose's Knitting Parlor and rented space to Dylan's Restaurant. He was renting office space on Eastern Avenue. Ro was a teacher at the Concord School. They lived in a big Victorian house on Railroad Street in St. Johnsbury. Trying to establish himself as a businessman and a business consultant, he was "working like a fool," he later said in an article in the

Caledonian-Record newspaper. In the fall of 2008, he had even run for office, competing in the Republican Primary for state representative from St. Johnsbury, but he had not secured the nomination. Then he got sick.

During the summer of 2008, Dennis was training for the November 1st New York Marathon. Somewhat pudgy as a boy, he had not been a school athlete, but he had always enjoyed hunting and in his forties had become a runner. As he had with earlier endeavors, Dennis was devoted now to running, fitness, and losing weight. He had competed in several marathons and shorter races, and was thin and fit. His training for the New York marathon had not gone well, however, so he had abandoned his plan to run it. In the fall hunting season, he had also felt weak and awkward in the woods and had fallen several times. In the winter of 2008 – 2009, he knew what the problem probably was. He underwent surgery for a double hernia in March but that did not improve his strength and coordination. He was diagnosed with ALS on April 21, 2009.

In July of that year, Dennis again asked for help from Habitat for Humanity, this time to widen his bathroom to make it wheelchair accessible. He was still walking and he talked with us as we worked. His breathing was labored, and I remember he leaned against the wall as he talked. At that time, I had not thought about writing this book, so I saw him as a sad case and a deserving Habitat client. Again, Dennis supplied all the materials so Habitat just supplied volunteer labor. Dennis's ALS was progressing quickly; by September of that year, he was on a ventilator.

On December 5, 2009, Dennis was the subject of a front-page article in *The Caledonian-Record*. "Businessman Fights ALS With Courage, Humor" was the headline, and Dennis was pictured sitting in a booth in his ice cream parlor, wearing a leather jacket, an ice cream sundae in front of him and a little smile on his face. His head was tilted to the side and a ventilator hose came out of his neck and around to the booth behind him. The same picture was used that fall in a "sexy" calendar published to raise money for ALS. The article told the story of the Farr family history, of Dennis's first symptoms and how they interrupted his career, and his intention to stay positive and contribute toward a cure. "Some days are cherries, some days are pits," he said in the article.

Mary said that back in February of 2007, before she retired, she had visited her primary physician, Dr. Sharon Fine, complaining of a twitching in her thigh muscles. Dr. Fine, she recalled, had brushed off the possible telltale symptoms of fasciculations, telling her, "I'm a lot more worried about the fact that you haven't had a mammogram in a while." Mary told me this story, and Hollis concurred: Mary knew all along that fasciculations, "tremblings" Hollis called them, were early symptoms of ALS.

Curiously, in light of the fact that the family has the fast-progressing A4V mutation, Mary carried on with her active life for two more years. Then in May of 2009 she experienced more definite symptoms of ALS while taking an aerobic exercise class. She was sixty-three years old at the time and had tried to assure herself that she was beyond the usual age of onset of symptoms of ALS. Her weakness and awkwardness had come on very gradually: first her left leg, then her left arm. She carried on with her life. She told me that she remembered walking on a beach in Maine with her friend Judy in June of that year and how unusually hard and tiring it had been. Her leg cramped, and she had found the stairs up from the beach to the bluff to be quite an obstacle. Then she had gone on a trip with a group of women friends in July and, again on a walk, someone had asked her, "White Top, why are you limping?" Mary met with Dr. Fine as soon as she got home on July 17. Mary was Dr. Fine's first ALS patient; although she had started her practice in Danville in 1997 and was aware of ALS in the Danville family. This time, Dr. Fine has said, when she examined Mary she knew she was looking at ALS.

Mary and Dr. Fine tried to get her an appointment at Dartmouth Hitchcock Hospital in Lebanon, New Hampshire, but were told that the earliest appointment that she could get with Dr. Elijah Stommel, the ALS specialist there, was in September. Mary asked Dr. Fine to mention that she was a member of the

Farr family, knowing that Dr. Stommel was aware of the family history and would certainly recognize that name; however the appointment secretary had repeated that September was the earliest possible date. Mary was upset at this.

She then got in touch with Massachusetts General Hospital and the office of Dr. Merit Cudkowicz. Dr. Cudkowicz immediately recognized the name and made an appointment for Mary in early August. At that appointment, Dr. Cudkowicz performed a few simple tests, and said to Mary, "Yes, you probably do have ALS."

Hollis recalled that Mary then said to him, "We have to start planning."

At that first appointment, Mary recalled, they talked about the family history and the research that Dr. Robert Brown had conducted to isolate the family's SOD1 gene. Mary agreed to be part of that study to further document the presence of the defective gene in the family.

Two days later, she heard from Dr. Cudkowicz by telephone confirming her diagnosis. Two days after that, Mary and Hollis made the three-hour trip to Boston again. She met with other members of the MGH neurology staff and agreed to be part of a trial of a new drug. Dr. Fine's notes of August 18 acknowledged that Mary's care was going to be largely in the hands of the neurologists, but she and Mary discussed her future needs, the progress of the disease, and even "briefly, end of life care." Dr. Fine urged her to complete an advanced directives form.

I first visited Dennis for this book on January 4, 2010. I had decided to take on the book project at that time, and began to visit both Dennis and Mary to learn firsthand about the disease and about the Farr family. Dennis was in a motorized wheel chair, which he could operate himself with the little muscle activity that he had left. He was attached to the ventilator, which was breathing for him through a soft tube placed directly into his trachea. He spoke in the rhythm of the ventilator; when it expelled air from his lungs he could talk, then he'd have to wait for the ventilator to fill his lungs before he could talk again. But he was anxious to talk and spoke constantly in that rhythm.

Dennis told me that he had decided to go on "the vent" (as patients call it) for two reasons: 1) he had a feeling that a treatment for ALS was close and perhaps he could actually benefit from it to prolong his life, and 2) his family's story was important to doctors. Perhaps he could contribute to the Farr's involvement in finding a cure for ALS. He was open, he said, to being part of any new treatment or trial.

He recounted his first symptoms for me. It was then that he disclosed that he had been feeling the symptoms back in 2008 when we had first met building the ramp. His father Charlie was present, and they began to fill me in on the family tree. Dennis described some of the difficulties of his first marriage. He thought that the family history of ALS had been one of the difficulties; in fact, he said, his wife's North Danville family had warned her about the family disease and urged her not to marry him.

In subsequent visits, Dennis described his career, updated me on his symptoms and the progress of the disease, and continued to tell me about his family. I met his wife Ro and their daughter Maura. On weekdays, Dennis was attended by Charlie and a health care worker. We talked about his care team, his family, and his circle of friends. His daughter Ashleigh had visited him and had even been part of his care team for a time.

His three brothers and his sister lived out of the area: Stephen in Martha's Vineyard, Massachusetts; John in Maine; Andy in central Vermont; and Cindy in Thetford, Vermont to the south. On a day-to-day basis, Dennis was visited by a small group of friends, notably Bob Butterfield and Bernier Mayo. Bernier would become Dennis's most loyal friend and champion during this time. A retired headmaster at St. Johnsbury Academy, Bernier is a devout Catholic. He visited Dennis several times per week, and would read to Dennis, sometimes pray, and was a constant and loyal friend. Every time I visited Dennis over the next two years, Charlie was there.

The big Railroad Street home had character, with its hardwood moldings, fireplace, and other details. It bespoke of elegance, but its elegance was in decline. Dennis's wheelchair was right next to a large picture window through which he enjoyed looking out onto the busy street. Driving down Railroad Street on nice days, I might also see Dennis in his reclining chair on his wide front porch, watching the traffic go by.

In the evenings and on the weekends, Dennis's care team was his wife Ro and his daughter Maura. They were devoted to him. The Myricks acquired a van with a ramp and lift, and Charlie, Ro and Maura learned to transport Dennis to get him out of the house. They would appear at church, at community and family events, and take Dennis to appointments. They took one trip to the Andrew Wyeth Museum in Farnsworth, Maine, and another to Camden, Maine, which Dennis had always wanted to visit. Charlie had a ceiling bracket installed in the bathroom of his cottage at Miles Pond so that Dennis could occasionally go there for a bath.

My first meeting with Mary Prior was in January of 2010 at the Danville Historical Society's newly acquired and remodeled colonial cape-style house on Hill Street in Danville. All subsequent visits were at Mary and Hollis's home, the same house first occupied by their nephew Curtis and Heidi in 1998. South facing from the top of a slope, with many windows, the home was filled with light and always neat and homey.

On most of the days I visited, Mary had either visitors or caregivers, or both. Her regular attendants were Hollis and friends and neighbors. Ellen Foster also cleaned the house for them. Terry Fairchild frequently spent time with Mary helping her complete the family history and genealogy. Neighbor Michelle Orr also stopped in and helped out. Mary also had home help from the area Home Health agency, the Vermont ALS Association, and an organization for ALS patients called Compassionate Care ALS.

Dennis and Mary both were accepted into a clinical trial for the drug Arimoclomol. Developed first in Hungary as a drug treatment for resistance to insulin and for diabetic complications, Arimoclomol had been acquired by the California pharmaceutical company CytRx in 2003 and was being developed and tested by CytRx for new uses. According to CytRx, Arimoclomol "is believed to function by stimulating a normal protein repair pathway through activation of molecular chaperones." According to a 2008 article in the *Journal of Neurochemistry*, it had been shown to be effective in mice with the SOD1 gene and symptoms. It improved their muscle function. It did so, the authors believed, by involving what they called the "heat shock response." In 2009, Arimoclomol was entering the phase II/III stage of the trial as patients began to get possibly effective doses. As participants in a double blind study, Mary and Dennis would not have known whether they were getting the drug or a placebo. Mary was also on the drug Rilutek; Dennis was not.

From the first of my meetings with Mary, she explained that she did not want to be a "poster child" for ALS. Over the years she had supported the efforts of her sisters Linda and Susan in their research into the history of the disease in their family, and in their fundraising and other efforts to help scientists find a cure for ALS, but as she explained it, she did not want be known only as a member of "that tragic family." Her marriage and family, her career, and her work with the Danville Historical Society and other community groups were the things for which she hoped to be remembered. Nevertheless, for as long as she lived with the disease, she was willing to be useful to the doctors; hence the enrollment in the drug trial.

Mary also made it clear that she did not intend to prolong her life by going on a ventilator that would breathe for her. When she could no longer breathe on her own, she intended to say goodbye. It seemed to me that, once Mary's diagnosis had been made official, she had quickly achieved a kind of resolve and peace, similar to that which her nephew Curtis had been able to achieve and which patients such as Franz Rosenzweig and Henry A. Wallace had found. Dr. Fine's notes of November 11 read, "She believes she is doing well. Her mood is upbeat. She feels that she has lots of support and is able to use it. She is enjoying life."

Mary was known for her honest and outspoken nature. She said what was on her mind, a feature that I would witness several times in the months that I knew her, and for which I would admire and grow fond of her. In our first meeting at the Historical Society, Mary was working with Sharon Lakey, who had already been chosen as her successor as director of the society. Mary had agreed to talk to me, but we kept getting interrupted. By coincidence, my sister Anne and her husband Art stopped to see an exhibit at the historical society, and Mary interrupted our conversation to give Art a piece of her mind. He, as chairman of the board of trustees of the Fairbanks Museum in St. Johnsbury, had recently participated in a difficult decision to separate the natural history collection and programming from the history and heritage collection. As a local historian, Mary opposed the split and she told Art so in no uncertain terms.

Hollis tells another story. Apparently it became known in the community that Mary had participated in ALS research by giving some of her body tissue, a patch of skin, for DNA research. That gave way to the idea that new tissue would be grown from that sample, which gave rise to the idea that the scientists, being neurologists, might grow another brain with Mary's DNA. A town selectman was heard to say, "My god, we don't need another Mary Prior brain."

On January 13, 2010, I received an evening phone call from Susan Lynaugh, Mary Prior's sister, who lived in the village of North Danville. At that time, Susan taught at Lyndon State College where I was a writing instructor. Susan is the first person from the Farr family whom I approached about writing this book. We had met regularly in her office at the college, over lunch, and she had begun the process of educating me about ALS and the family history. Susan had created a wondrous version of the family tree on butcher paper—color coded with pasted notes attached—which she had tacked up on her office wall for me to study during those sessions.

In the January phone call, Susan was very excited. On the previous day, she, her sister Linda and her brother Clif had traveled to Boston with Mary to meet with Dr. Merit Cudkowicz at Massachusetts General Hospital. A well-known and respected neurologist in the field of ALS and other motor neuron diseases, Dr. Cudkowicz was treating Mary, had entered her into the Arimoclomol trial, and was considering her for other clinical trials. Dr. Cudkowicz had surprised them that day, to some degree, because she was dressed more formally than usual, and she seemed particularly buoyant. The family members were there also to present Dr. Cudkowicz with a check from the Curtis Vance Memorial Orchard Foundation.

After the check passing and picture taking, however, Dr. Cudkowicz had told them that she had exciting news that she wanted to share. MGH had just received news of FDA approval of a clinical trial of a new drug. The drug she described as a "major medical breakthrough." It had "stopped" ALS in mice, and had the potential to even regenerate motor neurons in the brain and spinal cord. There were to be trials at four sites in the U.S, she said, and MGH was one. Dr. Cudkowicz had explained the three-stage process of clinical trials, and that the low-dosage trial just beginning was only for tolerability. She held out hope that Mary could join the trial in Phase Two, when the dosage could actually do her some good. There was hope that this was a development that could save Mary's life. In Dr. Cudkowicz's office there had been much joy and some tears, even from the doctor, Susan said, and she just had to call me and tell me about it.

The drug, to become known simply as ISIS-SOD1-Rx or ISIS 333611, was being developed by ISIS Pharmaceuticals of Carlsbad, California. It represented a new category of drugs called antisense oligonucleotide compounds, and would be administered in a relatively new way, to be injected intrathecally; that is, directly into the spinal fluid. Subjects recruited for the study would all be patients diagnosed with ALS and identified as carrying the SOD1 gene defect or mutation. As ISIS described the technology on its own website:

Antisense technology represents an important breakthrough in the way we treat disease. The explosion in genomic information led to the discovery of many new disease-causing proteins and created new opportunities accessible only to antisense technology. We have led the industry in the development of RNA-based technologies and successfully developed a drug discovery platform based on our antisense technology. We discover and develop drugs that bind to RNA instead of proteins, which have been the focus of the pharmaceutical industry for more than 100 years.

In an April, 2011 article about the drug and the technology in the MDA/ALS newsletter, SOD1-Rx was further described as "an antisense molecule directed against the genetic instructions (RNA) for the SOD1 protein." Antisense compounds, the article explained, are "pieces of genetic information that prevent other genetic information from being processed." The drug was designed to "reduce synthesis of the SOD1 protein." The drug trial was being supported by the Muscular Dystrophy Association and the ALS Association, and was taking place at six medical centers in the U.S. in La Jolla, Baltimore, Boston, St. Louis, Charlotte, and Houston. Primary investigators were Dr. Cudkowicz and Dr. Timothy Miller of Washington University School of Medicine in St. Louis.

Earlier studies, as Dr. Cudkowicz had reported to the family, had shown that ISIS-SOD1-Rx had "blocked production of SOD1 in the central nervous system and prolonged life in rats with a disease that mimics ALS." The idea of reversing the progress of ALS had caught the imagination of all involved, family and apparently doctors as well.

Susan had also said on the phone that night that the family felt triumphant in a way because its contributions to finding a cure for ALS had gone through MGH. They imagined that their family history, their funds, and perhaps some of their DNA, had gone into the research that had led to this drug. At this point I felt that this book could have a happy ending.

In March of 2010 at the Danville town meeting, Mary, from a wheelchair, argued vigorously for an appropriation for the Historical Society. In her presentation, she alluded to her illness. Danville voters, however, mindful of the need to hold taxes down during the recession, voted down the appropriation. I watched as several people, some of whom had argued and voted against the appropriation, stopped to say a few words to Mary—and most likely to hear a few words from her—as they returned to their seats after voting. I saw admiration and respect, even some affection, for the woman against whom they had just debated. After the vote was announced, someone from the citizenry gathered for the meeting called out, "We love you, Mary."

Early in 2010, I found that visiting Mary and Hollis was easy and pleasant. I would just stop in when I was in town. Often, there would be other family members or friends there helping out with Mary's care. In my talks with Mary, and in Dr. Sharon Fine's notes, I learned that as the muscle weakness and other muscular effects spread to other parts of her body, Mary began to draw a distinction between "frustration" and "anxiety." She was frustrated about her equipment and her inability to find comfort sitting in a wheelchair all day, or about the many adjustments she had to make in her awake and her sleeping routines, and the quality of care she was getting from the official support organizations. She confessed to Dr. Fine that she would take out her frustration on Hollis. But her mood in general, with the prospect of only months to live, Dr. Fine described as "upbeat." She was not anxious about her fate. She had come to accept it.

In the early months of 2010, as her symptoms worsened, Mary had two projects that she wanted to complete before she lost her abilities to do so. She worked conscientiously on a family history and genealogy, and she continued her tole painting. She painted beautiful designs, mostly flower petals, on trays, tin boxes, and wastebaskets. In most cases, she had a person in mind to whom she had promised an item, or to whom she wanted to give the piece. She did beautiful work. Today those pieces are prized items that help friends and relatives remember her.

In March, she and Dr. Fine discussed, and Dr. Fine wrote a prescription for, a gel seat for her wheelchair, and a Hoyer Lift. As of that visit in March, Mary was on no medicines for attitude or anxiety. Again Mary and her doctor discussed advanced directives, do-not-resuscitate orders, and several scenarios for the end of her life.

Early in April, I arrived to find a caregiver there from an organization called Compassionate Care ALS. Founded in 2003, according to its website, Compassionate Care ALS was originally the idea of ALS patient Gordon Heald. It was founded to provide equipment and home modifications specifically for ALS patients whose insurance coverage did not provide all they needed, such as home ramps, bath and shower chairs, and lifts. The Compassionate Care representative that day was John Sheeran of Sandwich, MA, a hospice chaplain and volunteer, who was providing Mary with a number of useful items: a back brace, a grabber, a hand ladder, and a belt to help others lift her.

Mary and John discussed what they saw as a "compassion gap." The medical profession, especially away from major ALS centers, was not really aware of the lives of patients and the everyday obstacles involved with movement, eating, transitions, and finding comfort, they felt. Even the ALS organizations—even the medical supply firms—didn't know how to teach patients to use the many devices they provided. Often, it seemed, they just dropped a device off and walked away, leaving the family to figure out how to use a wheelchair, a Hoyer Lift, or a medical bed. Compassionate Care's mission, John explained, was to give advice and to listen, sitting "eye-to-eye" with the patient. Even inns and public spaces supposedly made to be "handicapped accessible" were poorly designed, John said. John also provided Mary with a copy of the latest edition of a guide for patients and families.

By April, Mary's breathing was becoming much more difficult.

Dr. Fine prescribed a BiPAP machine. In a home visit, Dr. Fine's notes indicate, they had a "long discussion regarding progression and end-of-life care." While agreeing to try the breathing machine, Mary stressed that she did not "want to be ventilator dependent." By that visit, Dr. Fine was confident that Mary's wishes were well documented: "She has an advanced directive, she is a DNR [do not resuscitate] and is registering with the state registry." Dr. Fine's notes also indicate that she would be prescribing morphine and Ativan, and that Hollis would be educated regarding administration of those drugs.

By May, Mary had begun to use Ativan at nighttime to help with sleep. She was enrolled in hospice.

When I visited Dennis during 2010, his primary caregiver was his daughter Ashleigh. She seemed caring and efficient in tending to Dennis's needs: checking his oxygen levels, suctioning fluids from his mouth and lungs, and talking to him.

Beginning in late October of 2010, Dennis's primary health worker was Angela Zambon. Angela took an apartment upstairs in the Railroad Street home, where she lived with her daughter, and was Dennis's primary daytime caregiver. Formerly a Licensed Nursing Assistant, she had relevant medical training and experience. She would stay with Dennis until he went into the hospital with pneumonia in early July of 2013.

On April 8 of that year, 2010, Mary, her sisters Linda and Susan, her brother Clif, and Linda's son Chris went to an appointment with Dr. Cudkowicz at MGH. I was invited to go along. We all traveled together in Chris's well-appointed minivan. We stopped on the way down for breakfast at a Cracker Barrel Restaurant; Mary stayed in the van reading. The conversation on the way down was jovial, with the family recalling old stories, and picking on each other in a light-hearted way, the banter often initiated by Mary. But there was both worry and anticipation in the air, as the siblings—perhaps more than Mary—were clinging to the hope that Mary could still join the ISIS trial, and that she would get the drug, not the placebo, and that it would work.

At Mass General, Chris took the valet parking option and we helped Mary negotiate the transition from car seat to wheelchair. She was very anxious during the lifting and sliding, afraid that we would drop her. Upstairs in the neurology department, Mary met with Dr. Cudkowicz's residents Matt and Robert, filled out paperwork, reported to them on her current symptoms, and took a preliminary breathing test. We understood that Mary's respiratory capacity would be the determining factor as to whether she was strong enough to be part of the ISIS trial. Mary, ever the live conversationalist, bantered with the two young residents, identified Robert's accent (he was Australian), and told a very funny story about a woman in St. Johnsbury who had suffered the indignity of public, audible flatulence, which was apparently a concern of Mary's as she blew into the machine which measured her lung capacity. Then we all crowded into the office of Dr. Merit Cudkowicz.

Dr. Merit Cudkowicz is the Julianne Dorn Professor of Neurology at Massachusetts General Hospital at Harvard Medical School. The daughter of Italian immigrants, she grew up in Tennessee and Buffalo. She first came to Boston as an eighteen-year old undergraduate, attending Massachusetts Institute of Technology and majoring in chemical engineering. Dr. Cudkowicz became interested in neurology as a graduate student in Public Health at Harvard and has remained in Boston and in that field. Today she is the director of the ALS clinic at MGH and of the Neurological Clinical Institute there. She is also a founder and co-director of the Northeast ALS Consortium (NEALS).

When I first met Merit Cudkowicz with Mary and her sisters and brother in April of 2010, she was forty-eight years old, and a very busy clinician, conducting research, supervising residents, writing grant applications, and serving on numerous committees. Tuesdays were her clinic days, she told me, when she met with patients and residents concerning the various clinical trials she was supervising.

We all sat almost knee to knee in her small office as she quizzed Mary and showed her concern for Mary's condition. Dressed in tan slacks and a black top with a pearl necklace (not a white coat), Dr. Cudkowicz was patient, attentive and caring. They also discussed the future, modifications to Mary's home, and tentatively approached the issue of end-of-life care. I didn't realize the significance of it at the time but my notes say that Mary announced, "I'm going to get some morphine and Ativan when the time comes." Such talk made her sisters uncomfortable.

Dr. Cudkowicz gave Mary and the family an update on current trials for Arimoclomol and the ISIS drug, and acknowledged the Catch-22 that Mary was in. Because this clinical trial was only in Phase One, testing for safety, if Mary were to join the ISIS trial at this stage, she would be taking the drug (if she was administered it at all and not a placebo) at a very low dose. Mary would not be taking the drug at an effective dose. However, to wait for the Phase Two of the trial would probably mean that Mary's weakness would rule her out. Again, Dr. Cudkowicz had Mary blow into the spirometer as we all watched in some suspense. But Mary's lung capacity was already too weakened for her to be able to join the trial. It became pretty clear that there would be no miracle cure for ALS in time for Mary Prior to benefit. "It may be good for my family," Mary said with a level of courage and realism that the rest of us could not achieve at that moment.

We met Mary's youngest sister Jane for lunch, and talked mostly of other topics. Then we lifted Mary back into the minivan—again with Mary in a panic during the transition—and drove back to northern Vermont. The return trip was quieter as, I suppose, the realization sunk in.

In visits with Mary that spring, I found her increasingly debilitated and frustrated. Her breathing was more labored; she was moving toward going on the BiPAP machine to help with her breathing, which was especially difficult at night. She wasn't sleeping well. "We're all Hoyer now," she told me at one point, referring to the Hoyer lift, a mobile device for lifting and transitioning a patient.

In May when I visited, Mary was continuing with her painting (her right hand still functioned). She was sitting in a recliner, nearly horizontal, with the item she was painting on her lap. Her hand was covered with paint. I met her son Greg who was visiting and would be staying into June to help out. She offered me some chocolate banana bread, and often changed the subject from ALS to news in the village: a divorce, an arrest, a development at the historical society. By May 24, she was nearing the end of her Arimoclomol trial, not knowing whether she was on the actual drug but not feeling that it had made any significant difference in the progression of the disease.

On June 9, my visit was shortened by the arrival of Dr. Fine. Mary said she was happy to have me stay but Dr. Fine said they had things to talk about. As I was leaving, Mary pointed to a small pile of clippings and other information about ALS. "Those are for you," she said. I thanked her and looked them over as I went to my car: several clippings and the Mitsumoto book for patients. This was the last time I saw Mary. I learned later that she was giving things away to a number of people, part of her preparations for departing from us.

Dr. Fine's own notes for that day indicate that again they had a long discussion of end-of-life issues. Mary was taking Ativan with more frequency during the day "to calm her down," but still using the BiPAP only at night. Mary told the doctor that while she enjoyed the company, she had too many visitors during the day to continually use the breathing machine. Her voice was weaker. They discussed the hospital setting and Mary's desire not to end up there; Hollis was in on the whole conversation. In this visit and in a follow-up visit, Mary and her doctor and her husband discussed "palliative sedation." Dr. Fine noted that Mary was "currently not a candidate" for that, but that she was "having more episodes of sad times," and "feels ready to die." Mary was worried about Hollis, who was awake frequently during the night to care for her.

In Dr. Fine's June 25 visit, she found Mary "incredibly frustrated," and "feeling sad at times." She had begun using the morphine to help her with "air hunger." While visiting Mary, Dr. Fine called

Dr. Cudkowicz in Boston, who, according to Dr. Fine's notes, had "nothing further to add." The focus of this visit was "completely on end-of-life care, with comfort."

Dr. Fine would make one more home visit, only four days later. She found Mary to be "quite groggy," and to be having side effects from morphine and other drugs, trouble sleeping, trouble eating, and feeling that she was having too much company. She was taking another drug for anxiety. There were no notes about an end-of-life scenario, almost as if it had all been talked out.

On July 1, 2010, Dr. Cudkowicz came to Danville. I was invited to visit with her and the family and was to come to the orchard right after lunch. When I arrived, Linda was already there and was upset. She told me that Mary had already been taking morphine and Ativan, that she was very much in control of events, and that she was determined to end her life soon. Linda said that she didn't disagree with the idea of Mary having control over her own life at its end; it was just too soon. Linda, who had been through so much and who usually put up a very strong front, choked up as she spoke.

Dr. Cudkowicz arrived with Susan, and Clif, who had been haying nearby, arrived on foot. We toured the orchard as the family proudly showed the doctor the apple trees, the log home and future bed-and-breakfast under construction, and Joe Hallowell's welded apple tree sculpture. I snapped a photo of the family giving a check from the family foundation to Dr. Cudkowicz.

Dr. Cudkowicz had met with Mary and Hollis before coming to the orchard. She said that she had discussed Mary's options for the end of her life. She agreed with Linda—or didn't want to argue against the idea—that it was too early. "Let nature take its course," someone said. Dr. Cudkowicz explained that morphine and Ativan do not in themselves hasten the end—they are palliative, they are sleep aids—but there seemed to be an understanding that Mary was ready to let go and that the end would be days, not months away.

In the days and weeks to follow, there was also something else on the minds of the family; something that Dr. Cudkowicz had reportedly said when she met with Mary on July 1. "Your children will not have to go through this," she had reportedly said, referring to hopes for a cure. She had also visited Dennis in St. Johnsbury that day and had said something similar to Dennis.

At the orchard, I asked Dr. Cudkowicz if results from the ISIS trial might give Mary something to live for. She answered no. The trial had recently recruited only its sixth test subject, they needed eight for Phase One, and Phase Two was a long way away. So far, she said, the drug had proven to be tolerable in five patients taking it, but it was difficult to find enough test subjects when the pool was limited to patients already suffering from ALS who had the SOD1 gene defect and who were not too weakened by the disease. One of the roles of the family was to help MGH and other test centers recruit patients from among the far-flung Farr family descendants and other SOD1 families.

Two days later, on July 3, my family members were just about to head down to North Danville village for the annual Fourth of July parade and festivities (held that year on the Third because the Fourth was a Sunday) when I checked my email. A member of the Habitat for Humanity board had written to tell me that she wasn't sure that she could make our next meeting, that she would have to wait until she found out the date of "Mary's service." That was when I first learned that Mary had died.

We went to the parade where I first ran into Clif standing outside the little market of the Curtis Vance Orchard Fund. He confirmed that Mary had died the previous evening at Northeastern Vermont Regional Hospital, with only Hollis in the room. I also talked with Linda and Susan. They were both very sad but resigned. "That's just like Mary," Linda said, "calling the shots." Susan had the role of public address announcer that day, listing the floats, marching units, and all the children and grandchildren in costume in the little parade. She got through it, but then hastened in tears to her own home on the main street of the village. As she passed me, she could only say, "It's what Mary wanted."

Later, in conversations with Hollis and Dr. Tim Tanner, I

learned of Mary's and Hollis's struggles with the decision and the steps they took, with Dr. Tanner, to bring her life to a peaceful end. Dr. Tanner, the colleague of Dr. Fine at the Danville Health Center, had attended to Mary on July 1 because Dr. Fine was not available. Dr. Tanner told me that the decisions in Mary's case and the advice he gave her were not that difficult. That is, her situation met the ethical and legal requirements for beginning the conversation—with her and Hollis—about when and how to let go of her life. Those requirements: Mary was well-informed, the decisions were made slowly and with much thought, the medical profession had made its best attempts to prolong her life and alleviate pain, and her condition was indeed terminal. She was in fact being kept alive by her breathing apparatus. The ethical principle involved, he explained, was patient autonomy, her right to make an informed decision.

At one point, Mary and Hollis had contemplated staying at home, where Hollis would himself administer the drugs that would allow Mary to sleep peacefully, and then he would turn off the BiPAP machine that was Mary's lifeline. In the end, however, it was decided that to protect all and in order for it to go smoothly, it should be done in the hospital by trained personnel, under the watchful eye of the hospital's staff, and under the guidance of established hospital protocols. So on July 2 Hollis and Mary, after the home visit by Dr. Tanner, had gone by ambulance to the hospital.

There, in a hospital room, Mary was under the care of Dr. Mike Rousse, who was the doctor on duty that evening. Dr. Tanner was in contact with Dr. Rousse by phone. The nursing staff was informed of the plan, and some of them were upset. In a later debriefing, they expressed their mixed feelings about the end-of-life decisions. On the one hand, they understood the concept of patient autonomy, and they understood that Mary's life was coming to an end and that she was not able to breathe on her own, but it was nevertheless a sad and difficult decision. Mary's oft-stated intentions were unequivocal.

Mary's medical records show that she was administered the drugs Versed, an anesthesia, and morphine, which would have had the effect of suppressing Mary's drive to breathe. She went to sleep as her breathing continued with the BiPAP machine. Then the BiPAP was removed, her pulse checked, and she was pronounced dead. Hollis was the only family member present. He told me that twice, as Mary was going to sleep, she lifted her right arm and waved her hand from-side-to-side as if to say goodbye.

Mary Prior's funeral was held on July 10, a hot and muggy day with a light rain, eight days after her death. The church service followed a committal service for family only at the Danville Green Cemetery. For the funeral service, Danville United Methodist Church was packed; there were people standing on the stairs to the basement. The family occupied the first two rows on the left side and members of the Danville High School Class of 1964 sat on the right side.

Mary had planned the service with strict orders, ignored only in part, to keep the whole service to twenty minutes. She had chosen the readings and hymns and even written brief introductions for some of the pieces. Rev. Carol Borland began with opening remarks, which she suggested did not count toward the twenty minutes. Early in the service, we all recited the children's classic Sunday School song "Jesus Loves Me."

There were readings from Robert Frost, Margaret Mead, and Walt Whitman, and scriptural readings from the Gospel of Matthew, and from Galatians and Micah. A fifteen person choir from the church sang two anthems, and we all sang two hymns: "How Great thou Art," and "Amazing Grace." Printed in the bulletin and said in unison was a prayer attributed to Lucinda Campbell of the United Methodist Women: "Dear Lord, Let us take action on the things we have voted so many times to take action on and haven't yet started. Amen."

The service ended with the child's goodnight prayer, also said in unison, "Now I lay me down to sleep, I pray the Lord my soul to keep. If I should die before I wake, I pray the Lord my soul to take. Amen!" To many, the service seemed all too short to adequately celebrate Mary's life, but everyone agreed: that was what she wanted. In keeping with Mary's wishes, ALS was not mentioned during the service.

After the service, people lingered outside and enjoyed lunch on the green. Among those there to honor Mary was her cousin Dennis, lying almost flat in a medical chair, hitched up to his respirator. He was attended by Ro, Maura and Charlie. I stopped to talk with them. As I discussed the service with Ro and Charlie, and got an update on how Dennis was feeling, Dennis was patiently typing with his eyes. Eventually his computer spoke the words he had composed. "She always had a little wisdom," it said.

Dennis's choices and Mary's choices were different, but they represented two paths that are open for ALS patients world-wide. All ALS patients eventually die of respiratory failure, and many choose to let go of life when they can no longer breathe on their own or with noninvasive measures. That was Mary's choice. But a patient's death can be postponed by the invasive process of a tracheostomy and the insertion of a respirator. That was Dennis's choice. Both choices have their logic and their appeal, as well as their disappointments and downsides.

At Mary's funeral, Dennis—through his father Charlie—told me that he was being considered for an experimental procedure and trial of a "brain implant." This possibility gave Dennis the hope and the rationale for his decision to stay alive. It gave him a purpose for living. For the next eleven months it gave him hope. Then he would be entered into the trial and his brain wired with electrodes, which gave him a task, some work to do. To Dennis and his family it justified his decision to go on the respirator. He was contributing to medical science and the future prospect that someday ALS sufferers, their bodies incapacitated by muscle wasting, could nevertheless carry on their lives.

Ro, who could at that time still read Dennis's emotions, as well as his explicit messages, told me that day that Dennis was "all excited," both by the possibility of the BrainGate trial, and by Dr. Cudkowicz's words of encouragement about the ISIS trial. Ro pointed out that the noted neurologist had not said that Dennis's children "*May* not have to suffer," but had said "they *will* not have to go through this." From the point of view of Dennis and his close family, then, there were two reasons to hope and to stay alive and be aware of what the future may hold.

Dennis was wired for the BrainGate trial in June of 2011. He would live for another two years and two months after his cousin's death. During that time, Dennis saw a third ray of hope: he became convinced that the Arimoclomol dose that he was receiving in the trial of that drug was an effective dose, and was working. During the fall of 2010, after Mary's funeral, Dennis felt that he could see some movement in his heretofore inert limbs, including his left thigh and right thumb. He reported that to Dr. Fine in her September home visit. After earlier reporting that she saw "Really no antigravity movement in his extremities," Dr. Fine wrote in September, "He does have trace movement of right and left toes."

In her progress notes of November 30 of that year, Dr. Fine listed a total of eighteen prescribed medicines on Dennis's chart, including Arimoclomol, medicines for digestion and bowels, anxiety, blood thinners, and pain. Using words like "He thinks" and "He believes," she recorded Dennis's own perceptions that he was building muscle mass, and increased function, however slight. The Arimoclomol trial had ended, but Dennis continued to take the drug because he believed that it was doing some good.

As 2011 began, Dennis's condition was pretty stable. He was completely paralyzed, "locked in," as Dr. Fine put it, but still able to slowly, letter-by-letter type out a message. To visit him was to talk at him, it seemed, knowing that he was fully aware and able to comprehend, then perhaps to chat with Charlie and his caregiver, knowing that Dennis was listening. Finally his Dynavox computer would speak what he had been typing. He spent that winter believing that the Arimoclomol drug was having an effect, and very much looking forward to the BrainGate trial. Dr. Fine visited Dennis at home every two to three months. He was concerned that he would not be chosen for the BrainGate trial because his paralysis was so nearly complete.

Finally Dennis was admitted into the BrainGate trial and, in June 2011, he traveled to Massachusetts General Hospital for the procedure. The BrainGate technology and software are designed to pick up the brain's intentions and bypass the nervous system to control a computer or prosthesis. The surgical procedure that Dennis underwent in June implanted an array of electrodes—a four-millimeter square silicon chip studded with one hundred hair-thin microelectrodes—into his motor cortex, the part of the brain that controls movement. In an ALS patient, the underlying assumption is that the patient's brain is working fine; the problem lies in the circuitry in the brain and along the spinal cord that sends messages of intention to the muscles. The muscles over time have weakened, not due to diseases in the muscles themselves but due to their not being used, not being signaled to get to work. Thus they atrophy.

BrainGate subjects like Dennis, as I would observe in sessions once he returned home, are simply asked to think about movement, to form an intention. In one session I watched, the technician from BrainGate, who had come from Boston, asked Dennis to think about moving a cursor, shown as a white dot on his computer screen, to catch up with a red dot in a square on the screen. In another session, she simply asked Dennis to think about making a fist. Dennis's results never resulted in a dramatic show of movement, such as that demonstrated by a BrainGate patient on the CBS program 60 Minutes. In fact, the brain activity in Dennis's case was actually evaluated later by scientists at Brown University, but the sessions were very satisfying to Dennis. He was told that they provided very useful information to the BrainGate team.

The BrainGate team gave Dennis a lot of time and attention, especially considering that they had to drive to St. Johnsbury from Boston as often as once a week, usually staying overnight and spending parts of two days with Dennis. The sessions helped Dennis feel useful, broke up the tedium of lying paralyzed all day, and made him feel that he was contributing to science and to a treatment for ALS victims—or at least a way to bypass the paralysis. In her notes from her first visit to Dennis after the implanting of the BrainGate electrodes, however, Dr. Fine reported that Dennis's depression was worse, that the placement of the BrainGate array in Dennis's brain was "a little off" and therefore he was having difficulty communicating with the BrainGate computer, and that his caregiver felt that overall he was losing ground.

By October 2011, Dennis had developed a bedsore, and had been suffering from a fever and diarrhea. The family and his caregiver had been struggling with his feeding tube. The process of caring for Dennis, of watching for every possible symptom with almost none of the usual input from the patient, was constant and tiring. Breathing, skin issues, digestion, urine and bowels, conjunctivitis in his eyes, pain, fevers, lung and heart function were always being constantly monitored. Dennis had begun what would be almost a constant series of antibiotics for the rest of his life. To use Dr. Fine's terms, he was also not always "arousable," sleeping for much of the day. Dr. Fine's progress notes of November begin to show discussions with the family about palliative care, hospice care, whether it was useful for Dennis to participate in any more clinical trials, and what to do when communication with Dennis became impossible.

By the time of Dr. Fine's December visit, Dennis's med list had reached twenty-three. He was still very committed to the BrainGate trial; it was almost as if that was keeping him alive. His various fevers and ulcers had healed and he was more comfortable. Ro was still concerned about the loss of communication with Dennis, feeling that she had not had a really good conversation with Dennis about advanced directives, and nothing was in writing. In terms of end-of-life care, then, Dennis was still "full code;" discussions about what to do when it seemed the end was near were just beginning, and discussions with Dennis were becoming ever more difficult. As 2012 began, Dennis passed his twenty-ninth month on a ventilator, the family was trying to remain upbeat and BrainGate testing continued. Dr. Fine's visits were not that often, one in February, then none until May, when she noted that "things had been pretty quiet for the last three months."

One day when I visited during this time, I watched as Angela gave Dennis his morning coffee. Dennis's entire nutritional intake, of course, was through his feeding tube and so the enjoyment of food, its taste, aroma and texture, was almost entirely missing from his life, but Angela started his day with putting just a little coffee in a syringe and putting it on his tongue, just to give him the sensation. We all could read the enjoyment in Dennis's eyes.

In July, Dennis began to suffer what would turn out to be a series of pneumonias. He spent time in both Northeastern Vermont Regional Hospital and Dartmouth Hitchcock Medical Center, as physicians tried to find the right antibiotics for the pneumonia and a urinary tract infection. His trach was changed to give him more air, and he was given a bronchoscopy to examine his throat more clearly.

When Dennis was admitted to the hospital for the first time on July 3, Angela Zambon ended her service as his caregiver. It was during the summer and Ro and Maura, now out of school, and eventually a new caregiver, were there to care for him. Dr. Fine's notes of July 18, say that Dennis had recently signed a five-year commitment to work with BrainGate, and that he was excited about the plan. Despite setbacks, and the threat of pneumonia, he was not about to give up.

By the end of the month, however, pneumonia had returned, as well as pseudomonas, a species of bacteria, and another UTI. Dennis was hospitalized again, and doctors were finding that he was resistant to more and more of the antibiotics. The night before Dr. Fine's August 3 home visit, Dennis had spiked a fever of 101.5. Ro told the doctor that she would be addressing the issue of advanced directives with Dennis and with his deacon, Bernier Mayo. Dr. Fine in that visit asked Dennis a series of questions: would he want further antibiotics (Yes), would he want to be hospitalized again "if indicated" (Yes). Discussions with Ro and with Dennis about end-of-life issues continued five days later when again Dennis's fevers persisted.

Ro had made one last call to Mass General to see if there were any investigational treatments available for compassionate use. She was told there were none.

Dennis was brought to the hospital again on August 22. Dr. Mary Ready was on duty. The pneumonia had returned. Again he was treated with the escalating series of antibiotics, his fever subsided, and he was sent home.

Dennis was admitted to the hospital for the last time on September 1. As it happened, Dr. Tim Tanner, who had treated Mary Prior at the end of her life, was the hospitalist on duty that day. Dr. Tanner discussed with the family the fact that they were running out of antibiotics that might treat Dennis's various infections. It was clear to Dr. Tanner, as he explained to the family and Dennis, that there was no hope, no more possible treatment of the pneumonias; they were not going to go away. Dr. Tanner tried to converse with Dennis, watching for clear Yes or No responses, and decided that Dennis could give clear answers. Dennis agreed to stop the antibiotics.

The next day, Dr. Tanner asked Dennis if he wanted to consider withdrawing the ventilator; Dennis clearly answered No. Before the end of the day, Dennis's sister Cindy came to say goodbye, and his father Charlie visited him in the evening for what would turn out to be the last time.

By the next morning, September 3, when the same question was asked about withdrawing the ventilator, Dennis clearly answered Yes. The family—Ro and Maura—were there to confirm the definite response, as were two nurses and Ro's aunt Rosemary Murray. Also present in the tight quarters of the intensive care room were his daughter Ashleigh and his friend Bernier Mayo.

A distraught Maura protested, "Don't do this, Daddy!" Dennis's father, who had also expressed his disagreement with the decision to let go of life, was not there at the very end.

Bernier led the group in prayer, and then an intravenous drip was started with morphine and Propaphal, a sedative. Ro and Maura both held Dennis in the hospital bed as he slipped into a deep sleep. Then the respirator was turned off.

A service to celebrate Dennis's life was held on September 7, 2012 at St. John the Evangelist Church in St. Johnsbury. Attended by over one hundred people, the service included a full mass, hymns, recorded music and several speakers. Speakers included Laurie Barefoot of the BrainGate team, as well as Dennis's long-time friend Bernier Mayo, who helped conduct the service.

Singing was led by Janet Edmondson of St. Johns, and included traditional hymns "In the Garden," and "Amazing Grace." The recorded music included "The Impossible Dream" from Man of La Mancha, and Louis Armstrong singing "What a Wonderful World."

In contrast to the service of his cousin Mary, Dennis's service did include mention of the family disease. While his friends and family celebrated his life, they also acknowledged the family's history of suffering and death, and the constant threat of ALS. They were asked to join in the fight.

Those who attended the service received a copy of a tribute to Dennis and a poem, both written by Ro. The tribute read:

If I had to pick one word to describe Dennis, it would be passionate. Everything he did embodied so much dedication, emotion and perseverance. Whether tinkering on his clunky tractor (which he loved), training horses, painting his watercolors, studying for law school, running marathons or serving on many community boards, Dennis put his full effort into each endeavor with tenacity and his own style of getting things done.

As this monster of a disease took hold of him, he recognized not only his need to understand the disease, he was compelled to work with researchers to find a cure. Dr. Robert Brown from UMass, and Dr. Cudkowicz from Mass General Hospital are the movers and shakers of the ALS world. They have been working with our family (and our family genes) for years. Dennis also volunteered to be part of the BrainGate study led by Dr. Leigh Hochberg also from Mass General Hospital. Imagine people with paralysis being able to control their movements just by thinking about it . . . you will see it happening in the future. Dennis was part of this study for over a year and so proud he could make this contribution while being totally paralyzed himself.

As we say goodbye to Dennis let's remember not only the fond memories, the smiles and the good times. Let's remember this disease is ravaging our community. Let's reach out to these world renowned researchers and give them our support as we continue to fight this monster.

In lieu of flowers, friends, family and admirers were invited to make donations to the Curtis Vance Memorial Orchard Fund, or the North Danville Community Club.

Clinical Trials

For a patient diagnosed with ALS, there is a window of opportunity to find and gain acceptance into a clinical trial. In most cases, the eligibility requirements for a trial require the patient to be sick with the disease but not too sick, as the patient's symptoms are carefully measured and monitored. It helps to be near a major ALS center where the trial is taking place. In addition, the timing has to be right in joining a clinical trial when the trial itself is in a phase in which a possibly effective dose is being administered.

For a FALS family, the monitoring of clinical trials is part of the on-going search for a treatment or cure that may help the next member of the family who gets sick. Keeping in touch with major ALS centers or ALS associations, or checking clinicaltrials.gov, the family activist may be watching closely for news of the latest, much-anticipated trial.

Clinical trials are approved by the FDA and are closely monitored. In many cases, there are negotiations between phases, conditions to be met as set by the FDA, and numerous filings. It is quite a public process; patients, families, and their physicians can find out what trials are in what phases, and results must be posted.

Clinical trials are organized in three phases. After studies of the compound have been conducted in the laboratory and often in animals, the drug is ready for testing in humans. As spelled out by the National Institutes of Health, Phase One studies are conducted with healthy volunteers and their purpose is mostly to study the safe delivery of the drug at low doses. Side effects are watched for, as well as how the drug is metabolized and secreted.

In Phase Two studies, the dosage is usually raised and the focus now is on effectiveness: does the drug alleviate symptoms, or cause biological changes, or delay the onset of symptoms, or, in the case of a terminal disease like ALS, prolong life. In this phase the study will become randomized, controlled, comparative and double blind. Very precise procedures are followed. The participant in the study who is receiving the drug will be compared to a patient receiving a placebo or a different drug, and neither the patient nor his or her doctor will know who is receiving the active substance and who the inactive substance or placebo (hence the term double blind). Safety and side effects continue to be monitored. If the drug seems to be safe and effective in this population, the drug is approved for Phase Three.

Phase Three studies may lead to FDA approval, so there is much optimism among the pharmaceutical industry, clinical centers, and of course the ALS associations and patients when a drug is approved for Phase Three. In Phase Three the drug's effectiveness and safety are studied in more patients at different dosages, and sometimes in combination with other drugs.

In this era of "precision medicine" and genetic medicine, there is much discussion of whether the old model, described above, is suitable. If a drug seems to have been ineffective in most patients, or in the "average patient" after statistical analysis, but does seem to have been effective in some patients with different physiologies and pathologies, then does that constitute a failed study? Conversely, if a drug is proven effective in a small, carefully chosen group, then does it constitute enough sampling?

For ALS patients and others with terminal diseases, there is also an FDA procedure for what is called "expanded access" or "compassionate use" of a drug outside a clinical trial. A physician can file a clinical protocol if he or she can show that the risk of using the drug is less than the risk to the patient caused by the disease. In addition FDA rules do allow for "accelerated approval" for a drug which "allows promising treatments for serious life-threatening diseases to bypass costly, large-scale efficacy trials and go directly to market," according to *The Washington Post*. *The Post* was writing about an ALS drug whose manufacturers and some activists and patients considered promising, but which had only been administered in a very small trial.

As this book went to press, the subject of clinical trials and trial design was a major topic within the ALS research community. It was the subject of the keynote address at the 25th International Symposium on ALS/MND in December of 2014 in Brussels. There, in medical journals, and within the ALS associations there was much discussion and debate about safety, false positives, adequate sample sizes, reliable indicators, bio-markers, the lack of a robust productive disease model for ALS, the continued usefulness of mouse models, and endpoints.

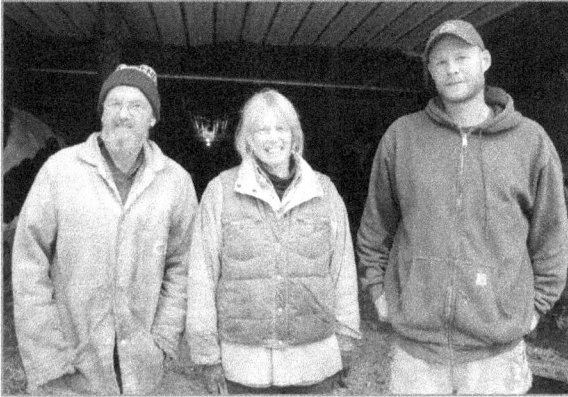

Clif Langmaid, Lee Beattie and her son Plynn at the farm,
North Danville village Spring 2014.

CHAPTER 8

Clif and the Ice Bucket Challenge

One year after the death of Dennis Myrick, in the late summer of 2013, as I was completing this manuscript (I thought), I was looking to get together with either Linda Vance or Susan Lynaugh, or both, to double check some of my facts and passages. I was having trouble getting through to them by phone, leaving messages that were not returned. I finally reached Susan, who seemed reluctant to talk about the book, and seemed generally sad over the phone. I should have been able to guess why. Finally, she agreed to meet with me a few days later.

Before we could meet, however, I managed to reach her sister Linda, who seemed equally reluctant to meet and talk and finally told me why: they feared that their brother Clif was showing symptoms of ALS. Clif was feeling a weakness in his right arm. They had made an appointment for him with Dr. Cudkowicz at Mass General for the next day, Friday August 30. I called Susan to postpone our meeting.

In the next few days I learned from a village neighbor of Clif's, and then from his nephew Craig, that their worst fears had been confirmed. Clif had revisited MGH on September 3 and the diagnosis had been confirmed: he had the early symptoms of ALS. Dr. Merit Cudkowicz had told him—as he later put it—that they "would throw everything but the kitchen sink" at the disease, that they would search the medical literature and find the most promising of clinical trials and get him into it. Based on the family's history with the fast-progressing version of the disease, however, he was told that he had better get his affairs in order, because he might not last a year. Clif was fifty-eight.

Clif Langmaid was the second youngest of the children of Forrest and Clara Langmaid. He was seven years old when his mother died in 1962. He was ten years younger than his sister Linda, eight years younger than Susan, and the only boy in the family. He had grown up without his mother. He helped out on the family farm as a young boy, showing an interest in farming, and after graduation from Danville High School in 1974, he attended Vermont Technical College and enrolled in its agriculture program. After graduating with an associate's degree from VTC in 1976, Clif returned to North Danville to help with the farm. After the death of his father in 1985, he took over managing the farm, the sixth generation to do so.

A slight, wiry man with a beard and mustache, Clif was quiet and hard-working, but always friendly, and like his father usually happy to stop and talk. This is the farm whose barn sits right in the middle of the village of North Danville. Clif managed the farm with its herd of high quality registered Holsteins. He never married, and ran the farm with his cousin Lee Beattie, his Uncle Phil's daughter, and in recent years her son Plynn. After the death of Clif's cousin Dennis in 2012, Dennis's brother John also had moved to the area and helped out on the farm.

After the death of his nephew Curtis in 1999, Clif was instrumental in creating the Memorial Orchard with his sisters Linda, Susan and Mary, helping with the landscaping and planting and tending the little orchard. But his main contribution, which became something like an obsession, was to build the large Apple Log Lodge. A two-story building made with logs of large diameter, the lodge is an impressive and beautiful structure, surrounded by extensive field stone walls and terraces laid by Lee's other son Phil. The lodge has a wide wrap-around porch, dormers, balconies and many windows, offering lovely views in all directions. With solar panels providing electricity, and large rooms, the lodge is offered as an attractive site for weddings or other occasions. It was definitely Clif's project, as he enlisted friends and relatives to help over the years with the next stage of construction. Once diagnosed, Clif wanted to complete the lodge as much as possible.

I met Clif four days after his diagnosis. He was parking his tractor when I was going by, so I stopped and he climbed out of the cab to talk. He showed me the weakness in his right arm, and was straightforward and brave, although unable to hide his emotions as he explained his situation. Once again, the family was putting its faith and future in the hands of Dr. Cudkowicz and her colleagues at Mass General. He used the "kitchen sink" phrase, and mentioned the case of a man who was in the news lately and had seemingly seen the course of the disease arrested. Clif seemed open to the idea of talking to me. He knew about the book, and we agreed to keep in touch. In that conversation, and in the days to follow, I noticed that it was Clif's intention to keep working as long as he could, learning to drive a tractor eventually with his left hand doing most of the work. I would pass him on the back roads or in the village and he would wave. He also was determined to keep the lodge project moving, that fall working to install the solar panels and batteries. Looking to find him for an update, I would sometimes find him at the orchard.

The man who had given hope to the world of ALS patients and families was Ted Harada of McDonough, Georgia. When diagnosed with ALS in May of 2010 at age thirty-five, Ted was married and the father of three. He had worked in the parcel post delivery industry and recently for a document shredding company. He entered a clinical trial at Emory University in March of 2011.

Patients in the trial were injected with 500,000 stem cells derived by the Rockville, Maryland company Neuralstem. The trial's leading investigator was Dr. Eva Feldman at the Taubman Institute of the University of Michigan. Although several other patients had seen the progression of the disease more or less halted, Harada's ALS had actually reversed. His symptoms had diminished; he no longer walked with a cane or had trouble breathing. With continuing weakness on his left side, he did not consider himself cured, but he was resuming a normal life.

Clif's MGH doctors, however, did not enroll him in the stem cell trial (MGH was not designated as a test site), but instead enrolled him in a small and short-term trial of immune-suppression drugs. It turns out that the subjects in Ted Harada's stem cell trial had also been given a regimen of immune-suppression drugs, including prednisone, to guard against the body's rejecting the stem cells. Dr. Jonathan Glass and his colleagues at Emory and other sites wanted to learn whether the "novel immunosuppression regimen" used in the stem cell trial was responsible for Ted Harada's "clear improvement." In a video that Harada had posted on YouTube, he could be seen playing wiffle ball with his kids, walking briskly down the street, and climbing stairs easily. He was even retested to substantiate that he indeed did have ALS. His case was the Farr family's latest hope.

Clif was first given the five-drug cocktail in September of 2013, and as the weeks went on the treatment seemed, from my own observations, to be slowing the progress of the disease. I would see Clif at events, or at work, or at his home, and while he kept his right arm at his side or in his pocket, he seemed to have full use of his left arm, walked well, and seemed to have no bulbar symptoms in his breathing or speech. To help with the haying that fall, his nephew Craig, Linda's son, invested in some extra equipment with funds from the family business, and neighbors, family and friends all pitched in. At the funeral of his uncle Arnold (his father's brother) in January 2014, he was circulating and chatting and reminiscing like everyone else.

As a form of family and community support for Clif, his sisters and he began to host regular Friday night potluck dinners at the Apple Log Lodge. Made known by social media posts and word-of-mouth, the dinners were open to everyone. Mounds of food would be laid out, and there were beverage and dessert tables. Using the lodge's two big rooms on two floors, the dinners accommodated as many as a hundred people, milling around talking in small groups. There was a lot of laughter and conversation. Clif might be holding court seated deep in an armchair one minute, then on his feet milling around the next. His sisters explained that the dinners meant a lot to him, and they provided friends and family a way to support him and his family yet again in their collective and continuing fight against ALS, without actually talking about it.

When I attended one of the dinners in May, nine months after his diagnosis, Clif took me aside and gave me an update, confirming that it was the immune suppression trial that he was in and that it seemed to be holding off the disease. To me, it looked like there had been little change since we first met four days after his diagnosis in September. In talking about the disease that evening, however, and in later visits, Clif was realistic; he could feel a general loss of strength and began to have a little trouble breathing and talking. His voice, never loud or deep, was becoming weaker.

In retrospect, his sister Susan told me, Clif began to live for those Friday night dinners, and wanted to make people comfortable by circulating among them while hiding his symptoms. He would rise to that occasion each week, literally, pulling himself out of his recliner to go to the lodge, then collapsing back into it afterwards. Clif was losing weight. It turns out that the major side effect of the immune suppression drug cocktail was an upset stomach. Clif and other patients in the trial found it hard to keep food down, lost their appetite, and could not get enough nutrition, adding to the weakness caused by ALS. It was later learned, according to his sister Susan, that some patients in the trial dropped out for that reason. As many ALS patients do, Clif began to spend his days in his recliner. Lee was his main caregiver.

In June, when I visited him at home, he was in his recliner. A breathing machine was on a table nearby, but Clif was not using it during the day. I was encouraged to see the positive effects of the drug trial, as it looked to me that—now ten months after diagnosis—Clif's ALS had not noticeably spread to his lower body. His left arm was showing weakness but was still useable, and I could not see or hear a lot of change in his breathing or voice. I had sat with Clif's sister Mary and his cousin Dennis, and ten months after their diagnoses, each of them was having significant problems breathing. Dennis was on a ventilator. After a pleasant talk with Clif and Lee, as I started to leave, Clif stood up from his recliner and showed me to the door.

At the annual celebration and fundraiser at the Curtis Vance Memorial Orchard on June 21, Clif was on his feet and very much at the center of attention. It was especially poignant, and a reminder of the family history, to have him there. During the charity auction, he was not able to occupy his usual role as an assistant to the auctioneer, his nephew Craig, holding up the next item and searching the crowd for bidders, but he was seated in the back center of the half-circle of bidders and spectators, often just quietly saying, "Thank you," for a particularly generous winning bid. He was also walking and talking on July 4th at the North Danville celebration.

One month later, however, on August 4 when I checked in with Susan, she told me that Clif was in Mass General. He had gone there for an adjustment to his medicines and to see what could be done about his continuing stomach discomfort and his weight loss. The hope on that day was that Clif would "fatten up" on IV fluids, adjust his medicines and return home to North Danville. Clif stayed at MGH longer than planned.

Clif and Lee had talked about his end-of-life preferences. They had coined the term "Orchard Day" to refer to that day when Clif would signal that he had had enough. After returning home from Boston, according to Lee, he did not feel any better, and was not able to sleep well or breathe without his machine. He was also very anxious. Early in the day on Thursday, August 7, Clif turned to Lee and said, "I think it's Orchard Day." He was taken to Northeastern Vermont Regional Hospital where he passed away that afternoon at about 5:30 surrounded by his family.

Clif's memorial service was held at his beloved Apple Log Lodge on August 13. Visiting hours were offered at the Lodge on the 12th and the 13th. The family buried Clif with a short ceremony at the Danville Green Cemetery. Once again, family and friends gathered to say goodbye to another member of the family. Donations were welcomed in his memory to be directed to FALS research at Massachusetts General Hospital.

The illness and passing of Clif Langmaid seemed to add an extra burden, almost an unbearable one, to the Danville members of the family who had now seen three members of that generation die in four years. The sadness was pervasive and inescapable, especially for his sisters, who expressed a feeling of extreme emotional fatigue. "I'm just so tired of losing people I love," said Linda. Earlier losses had been spaced years, even generations, apart. Several cases of FALS had been masked by other symptoms or explainable by old age, or had occurred in another state, or in some way had spared the family the horror of realization and close experience, the pain and fatigue of caregiving, and the witnessing of the wasting away of a loved one. The loss of Clif, a sweet, hard-working, man of fifty-nine years, was almost too much to bear.

· · · · ·

It was right about the time of Clif's death, early August 2014, that the ALS associations began to notice an uptick in donations, and realized the phenomenon which came to be known as the Ice Bucket Challenge. The social media fund-raising phenomenon began in the early summer when a group of golfers, including Greg Norman, and a motocross racer began to use social media to show them dumping a bucket of ice water over their own heads and challenging others to do the same. The typical challenge was to dump the ice and donate ten dollars to one's favorite charity or skip the ice dunking and contribute one hundred dollars.

The original charities did not include ALS. When NBC's Matt Lauer doused himself on *The Today Show* on July 15, he pledged to donate to a hospital, but on the same day a professional golfer named Chris Kennedy took the challenge and he in turn challenged his wife's cousin who challenged an ALS patient named Pat Quinn who challenged another ALS patient named Peter Frates. That's when the social media challenge went viral and the idea was appropriated by the ALS community. Soon it was known as the ALS Ice Bucket Challenge.

Peter Frates, a former Boston College baseball player, was diagnosed with ALS in 2012. He is well connected in the ALS community. He is affiliated with the ALS Therapy Development Institute in Cambridge, Massachusetts, and was on the Charlie Rose Show as part of Rose's series on the brain. Frates has a huge social media following. Once he issued the challenge on July 31, it took off. Soon it seemed everyone on Facebook was taking a video of himself or herself getting doused with a bucket of icy water, then challenging particular friends or acquaintances to do the same or pay up. It reached Danville soon after Clif's death, as dozens of friends and family in his memory took the challenge and wrote a check.

The national level of awareness of ALS received a great lift from the Challenge, as did the reality of familial ALS. One of the most moving videos of someone taking the ALS Challenge was that of Antonio Carbajal of Riverside, California. In addition to his own dunking, and footage of himself dressed in a pink bikini and washing his car, his video shows Carbajal caring for his mother, who has ALS, and his tearful revelation that he too has been diagnosed with the disease.

In Danville the awareness of the special case of the Farrs resulted in a community event. On Sunday September 21, hundreds of people turned out on the Danville Green for food, music and a mass dousing. A table was set up to accept donations, to be forwarded directly to Massachusetts General Hospital. The newspaper the next day estimated that over a hundred people took the challenge, having brought their own buckets, after a count-down lead by Hollis Prior. Linda Vance was pictured in the newspaper with a bucket on her head. For a bucket she used one painted by her sister Mary Prior in her last days. According to organizer Kitty Toll, the event raised more than $10,000 for MGH, added to over $32,000 that had been donated by the small community in recent months at the auction in June, in memory of Clif, and in previous Ice Bucket challenges.

In the months to follow, the various ALS associations and research centers each reported on the amazing windfall of donations, and on their plans to make good use of the funding. By mid-August the ALS Association reported that it had received over $160,000 in contributions over a ten day period compared to donations of $14,480 during the same ten days of the previous year, but that was just the first wave. Soon that figure had grown to $2.3 million and, counting local chapters' receipts, over $4 million. By September 22, the ALS Association was reporting a total of $115 million, and by April of 2015 reporting over $200 million worldwide. The ALS associations and centers began setting up meetings and forums to decide how to best spend the money.

The various research centers such as at MGH and ALS TDI also began posting their numbers and their intentions. By the end of August the ALS Therapy Development Institute was reporting over $3 million in donations itself and announcing its intention to expand its precision medicine program to enroll hundreds of patients compared to its previous goal of twenty-five (see discussion in Chapter 9). Mass General's Dr. Merit Cudkowicz announced that with $10 million from the Challenge and using new imaging technology from General Electric, MGH planned to study more closely the effects of ALS on the brain. Drs. Michael Collins and Robert Brown of UMass Medical Center took the challenge in white coats on August 22 and challenged executives at Biogen Idec to do the same. A *New York Post* article named Biogen Idec and Isis Pharmaceuticals as two of the drug companies most likely to benefit from the sudden influx of funds.

In addition to raising funds, the Ice Bucket Challenge raised awareness of ALS. The "orphan disease" was all over the media and stood to be adopted by wealthy donors and other caring people. Local associations and their events reported greater participation. Wealthy donors provided matching funds, and the total ballooned. By October the ALS Association announced its initial plan to spend $21.7 million, along with a matching donation of $12.5 million, for a total of $34.2 million to support six programs. Among the six programs were the Accelerated Therapeutics partnership for a "multi-pronged approach to expediting clinical trials," The New York Genome Center for understanding the genetic bases of ALS, The Neuro Collaborative of California to develop antisense therapies for the C9orf72 gene and gene therapy to down regulate SOD1, and Project MinE's global effort to sequence the genomes of at least 15,000 people worldwide with ALS.

The ALS Association and its state and regional affiliates also weighed whether to invest in research or to supply more funds for patient care. Always a balancing act, the various associations and support organizations struggle to divide their available funds between an investment in the search for a future cure, and direct present help for those afflicted with the disease. The Ice Bucket Challenge enabled the ALS Association to double its annual grants to forty-three Certified Treatment Centers across the United States, for a total of $1.075 million.

PART V
The Future

The Promise of Genetics:
Going to be Tested

The words in nearly every obituary, "He/she is survived by..." have a different meaning for families with familial ALS. The patient's struggle is over but the family curse remains. The arrival of symptoms in a sibling or parent carries with it a message to their kin—I could be next—and leads to a series of choices and decisions to be faced and made, or (in many cases) to be deferred or ignored. The family tree tells an individual family member that he or she has a chance of contracting the disease and a chance of being a carrier and passing on the gene and the disease to a child. Today there is the possibility of knowing whether or not you carry the gene.

If a person has a family history of ALS, and prior testing of the family has identified the particular defective gene, then that person could be a candidate for genetic testing. The testing, called presymptomatic testing, will determine whether this individual has the particular defective gene. The test begins with giving blood to a licensed, specialized lab, and it takes two or three months to get the results. The test costs from $300 – $4,000 depending on how many specific gene tests are to be done.

Genetic testing for FALS is preceded and followed by counseling with a certified genetic counselor. There is a lot to think and talk about. According to genetic counselor Lisa Kinsley of Northwestern University's Neuromuscular Disorders Program, the pre-testing session is very important. All members of the family are welcome to attend this session, and there is a set protocol of topics to be covered. The session accompanies a basic neurological exam, and the family history is reviewed. All topics, all the what-ifs, are reviewed at this time so that the family can decide if they want to be tested, and so that they will be prepared to handle the results. In the case of an autosomal dominant inheritance pattern such as SOD1, a coin flip is a good analogy, counselors say. The test is the coin flip; it will come up heads or tails, but for four siblings it could come up heads four times. It is important, Kinsley stressed, that there are no surprising medical facts, or possible outcomes, revealed after testing. All odds and eventualities need to be on the table. The counseling is a very delicate process, with psycho-social as well as clinical considerations, and the counselor needs to play it by ear. He or she needs to gauge the patient's and family's reactions at each stage.

In some cases, a family member may decide in that first session to go ahead with the testing and blood will be drawn. In other cases, they may want to think about it, because once the testing is done there is another tough decision to make: do they want to know the results? Sometimes, according to Kinsley, an FALS family member may decide not to give blood for testing, not to have any more counseling. Sometimes, they cancel the second appointment. Sometimes, they simply are no-shows.

Once the results are available, there is another counseling session. Again, close family is invited. Again, the patient can decide not to know. It is protocol, however, when the client is ready, to reveal the results early in the session, not asking the FALS member to wait. Then, the implications, the possible scenarios, and the various odds are all reviewed.

The benefits of genetic testing are limited by two facts: 1) there is no cure for ALS, and 2) there is no certainty about age of onset, or whether the client will even get symptoms. A family member who tests positive for the SOD1 gene defect may still be one of those people who never get ALS (they are called obligate carriers), or may have symptoms late in life, and if they do there is currently nothing that can be done to treat it. Once a positive test is revealed, telling him or her that they do have the gene defect, there is also nothing that can be done to prevent or delay the onset of the disease.

In addition, a person who tests negative for the SOD1 gene defect, while feeling a great sense of relief, and a freedom to plan for a good long life, may feel "survivor's guilt," or regret past decisions based on presumed risk, or "find it hard to let go of that part of their identity." If you are a Farr, for example, you are a member of a well-known clan with a certain identity tied to family history. Testing negative puts you on a "safe" branch of that family, and it allows you to go ahead and have children, if you had been undecided, or to make other choices, but it is never comfortable. Several Farr family members have said to me, "I wish it had been me," or "It should've been me."

As a member of the clinical team at Northwestern, Kinsley is already familiar with the families, their history, and even the lives and deaths of past family victims. The Northwestern Neurological Disorders Program is to certain Midwestern families what the Mass General program is to the Vermont Farrs: their connection to the world of advanced ALS science and to any kind of hope. The Northwestern staff members have their own Farrs.

Genetic counseling and testing centers also offer prenatal testing. Again, if the disease-causing defective gene has already been identified in the family, and a young woman knows that she and any future children are at risk for ALS, she may submit fetal cells, obtained by amniocentesis or by chorionic villus sampling, for DNA testing. According to genetic counselors, this procedure is rare and is undertaken only with careful consideration of the choices facing the parents. A positive prenatal test for the SOD1 gene or another FALS gene leads to very difficult decisions about termination of the pregnancy. Prenatal testing of fetal tissue could also reveal the mother's genetic makeup, if she has not previously been tested herself.

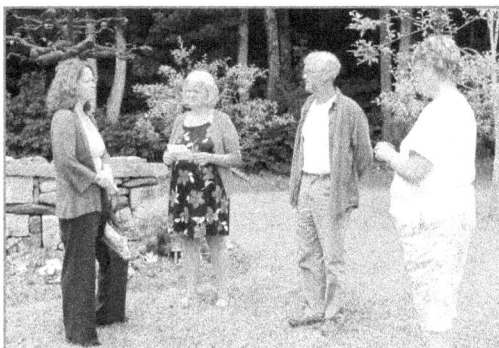

*Dr. Merit Cudkowicz, Susan Lynaugh, Clif
Langmaid and Linda Vance at the Curtis Vance
Memorial Orchard July 2010.*

CHAPTER 9

Hope and Defeat,
Advances and Setbacks

Amyotrophic lateral sclerosis is a so-called orphan disease. That is, it affects relatively few people, and once
affected they don't live very long. As spelled out bluntly in the
Rare Disease Act of 2002 law, "Such patients were denied access to
effective medicines because prescription drug manufacturers could
rarely make a profit from marketing drugs for such small groups of
patients. The prescription drug industry did not adequately fund
research into such treatments. Despite the urgent health need for
these medicines, they came to be known as 'orphan drugs' because
no companies would commercialize them." As defined in the 2002
revision of the original 1983 law, a rare disease is any disease that
affects less than two-hundred thousand people at any given time.
ALS, Huntington's disease, Tourette syndrome, Crohn's disease,
cystic fibrosis, cystinosis, and Duchenne muscular dystrophy, are
given as examples in the law. The law counts six thousand of these
diseases, affecting twenty five million Americans.

In sporadic cases when an individual is diagnosed with ALS, he or she and his or her family and loved ones have perhaps two years to get acquainted with the disease and search the world for some sort of new treatment. In families with a history of the disease, the search is on-going, as family activists monitor the latest trials and therapy ideas hoping for a promising development before the next member of the family begins to show symptoms. In the fall of 2012, when Dennis Myrick died, there was little medical news that families could grab on to, but they held on to hope.

On November 1 of that year, I attended an ALS "Leadership Summit" sponsored by the ALS Therapy Development Institute (ALS TDI), a unique, nonprofit, pre-clinical organization for the study of ALS and the search for a cure. At the summit held in a Boston hotel, neurologists and representatives of drug companies, research labs, charitable foundations, and patients and their families—all of the stakeholders in the fight against ALS—gathered to hear the latest. In the morning, we heard from representatives of two pharmaceutical companies and from Steve Perrin, CEO and Chief Scientific Officer of the ALS TDI about specific promising directions for therapy, and from Dr. Robert H. Brown who provided an update about advances in studying genetic pathways. After lunch, there was a panel discussion featuring two representatives from the pharmaceutical industry, a foundation executive, a journalist, a representative from the NIH, and Perrin, followed by questions and answers.

The morning presentations were all illustrated with PowerPoint presentations, most of them showing charts and graphs, bullet points, and slides and short videos of SOD1 mice. Each presenter explained the theory behind his or her therapy, and the published results of studies and trials. They respectfully acknowledged each other's science, while politely alluding to slight disagreements. In his opening remarks, Steve Perrin of ALS TDI referred to the day's presentations as a "view from 10,000 feet of the state of the union" on ALS, and mentioned seven promising directions for developing compounds for treatment that ALS TDI was monitoring.

Mentioned several times was the soon-to-be completed Phase III trial of a drug developed by pharmaceutical giant Biogen Idec.

The drug, dexpramipexole, had shown efficacy in the Phase II clinical trial, both slowing symptoms and extending survival times. So Biogen Idec had extended the trial to the relatively rare stage of Phase III, the last stage before FDA approval. There was much hope among scientists and patients, but at the Leadership Summit, the expectations seemed muted; none of the scientists, clinicians, patient advocates, or fundraisers on the panel extolled the drug.

Toward the end of the day at the Leadership Summit, during the panel discussion, a woman in a wheelchair, raised her hand and asked the panel members to "look into your crystal ball" and give families some reason to hope. The panel members each looked to their right and left to see who was going to provide an answer, then one-by-one they offered careful responses. Dexpramipexole was mentioned. The energy booster creatine was offered, as well as the possibility that a drug which has proven effective for another disease, such as Multiple Sclerosis, will prove to be effective for treating ALS.

"I feel that something will happen very soon," said a pharmaceutical representative. "There are over 140 drugs in development," but the questioner's face did not register hope or excitement in response to anything that anyone had said.

Diseases are in competition with each other for the millions of dollars expended or invested by the National Institutes of Health, and by pharmaceutical companies, large private foundations, private investors and venture capitalism firms, medical centers, universities, small family foundations such as the Curtis Vance foundation, and wealthy caring individuals. In this competition with other diseases, ALS has both strengths and weaknesses in its appeal. Its weaknesses:

The Numbers

Both the incidence and prevalence of ALS are low. It affects very few people—only about five thousand cases per year in this country—and, due to the relatively quick progress of the disease, the number of Americans affected by ALS at any given time (the prevalence) is only about thirty thousand. As a result, a pharmaceutical company that created an effective drug would have only thirty thousand potential US customers at any given time, and perhaps three hundred fifty thousand worldwide.

Poster Children

In addition to there being relatively few victims, there are very few child, young adult, or even young parent victims. A poster child for the disease will not usually be a child. Most sufferers from ALS are in their forties or fifties and they are usually not clustered in any geographical, demographic, or occupational way. Ninety percent of ALS cases are of the sporadic kind.

Since Lou Gehrig, there have been a number of celebrity patients struck down while in the public eye. There have been many well-known victims who have been public about their diagnoses and life with the disease, but because of the relatively quick and inexorable progress of the disease, they don't remain in the public eye as victims for long. Further, because the disease eventually affects speech, they are not able to be spokespeople for very long.

The face of ALS is male. Almost all of those listed on the various lists of notable people who have had ALS are men. Although ALS affects men only slightly more frequently than women, only three women are included on the list of notable people who have been affected by ALS as posted by the ALS MND (Motor Neuron Disease) Alliance. The ALS MND list does not include Broadway producer Jenifer Estess. Diagnosed in 1997 at age thirty-four, Estess testified before Congress in favor of expanded stem cell treatments in 2000. She and her sisters started a foundation to raise money for the search for a cure. They called it Project ALS. Estess wrote a book, appeared on talk shows, and made a documentary for HBO. She died in 2003 at age forty.

The Sad Treatment History

Seventy-five years after Lou Gehrig's diagnosis, there is but one relatively ineffective drug for the treatment of ALS. There are virtually no ALS "survivors" to tell their stories. Although there is much activity, more ALS centers in major hospitals and universities, and constant clinical trials, there has been no major break-through. At the start of 2015, there was no promising Phase III clinical trial underway. Recent statements by prominent doctors have emphasized that the disease poses a very complex picture. A cure or treatment will be "multifactorial," they say.

The Media's View

As compared to the shaking palsy of a Parkinson's disease patient, the pale cancer victims without hair, a heart patient clutching his chest, or a lung patient gasping for breath, the image of an ALS patient may be less clearly implanted in the public consciousness. ALS symptoms are not bizarre physical or verbal manifestations, such as those of Huntington's disease or Tourette syndrome. The disease manifests itself as a quiet, sad immobility. There is Gary Cooper as Lou Gehrig speaking at the mike, there is Stephen Hawking slouched in a wheelchair, there is former Massachusetts Governor Paul Celluci in a chair, pictured on a billboard. The common view of the ALS patient, by my guess, is what viewers of the 2013 NFL draft saw on television when former New Orleans Saints player Steve Gleason wheeled himself on stage to announce the Saints' latest pick. With his much-reduced size, his long hair cut short, and his once powerful arms and legs withered and immobile, he hit a button to start the prerecorded message that revealed the Saints choice in the third round. He managed a small grin as his own voice, synthetically recorded, announced the pick.

The common view of ALS is that it is sporadic, as few members of the general public are aware of the inherited form; no celebrity patients have been FALS patients. Families with a history of the disease, such as the Farrs, are known within their communities but not to the world. This fact was altered somewhat during the phenomenon of the Ice Bucket Challenge in the summer of 2014, as several videos of ice dumping went viral and several featured FALS patients.

The prominent ALS patient pretty quickly disappears from public view. Before long he or she cannot walk, talk, or shake hands. Michael J. Fox, in contrast, has been the face of Parkinson's disease for twenty-one years, and is still acting and speaking.

· · · · ·

The ALS community of patients, their families and their doctors, however, also have their case to make. When they try to raise funds or encourage medical scientists to engage in the search for a cure, the perceived weaknesses are turned into strengths:

The Numbers and Orphan Drug Special Status

As a designated orphan disease, ALS has a special status as first specified in the Orphan Drug Act of 1983. Since the passage of that law and in amendments since, pharmaceutical companies and other drug development organizations pursuing treatments for orphan diseases have a number of incentives: 1) they have access to government subsidies for research, 2) they can achieve tax breaks, and 3), most importantly, they can acquire extended patent protection rights and a seven year exclusive right to market the drug once it is approved by the FDA. They can also charge more for the drugs. The 1983 act created an Orphan Products Board within the Department of Health to oversee the program.

Poster Adults

While a single representational figure for ALS has not emerged since Lou Gehrig, certain profiles have emerged for a time and perhaps gathered in the public mind. What the disease has done to certain prominent people, robbing them of their ability to display their particular talents, has for a time caught the attention of a sympathetic public. There seem to be several of these profiles.

There is the **philosopher**. In 2010, Terry Gross of National Public Radio interviewed the historian Tony Judt, who at that stage was much weakened by ALS. Judt spoke in the slow, measured language of the patient on a respirator, seeming to pause to gather his thoughts as well as his breath. Philosophical, amazingly open and analytical about his own case, Judt revealed the same qualities and mindset as those of philosopher Franz Rosenzweig or Henry A. Wallace—the philosopher-patient. Judt was sixty-two years old at the time and would die in August of that year. Other prominent thinkers and academics who have shown the effects of ALS and in the process presented a portrait of the brilliant mind encased in an unresponsive body, include Morrie Schwartz of Mitch Albom's hugely popular *Tuesdays with Morrie*; Fokko du Cloux, Dutch mathematician and computer scientist; and theoretical physicist Stephen Hawking. For as long as Hawking has been known by the general public as a cosmologist, he has also been known as an ALS patient, perhaps the most famous, recognizable case of the brilliant mind encased in a wracked body. Hawking, whose case is unusual in its slow development, has appeared in television sitcoms, even a British commercial, and was featured in the movie *The Theory of Everything*, released in 2014.

There is the **athlete**. In his excellent PBS series on the brain, Charlie Rose brought together a panel to discuss ALS and other disorders of the motor neurons. In his July 2012 television broadcast, the ALS patient at the table was Peter Frates of Boston, a former Boston College baseball player. At age twenty-eight, Frates was handsome, articulate and noble. He showed few symptoms at that stage, shortly after his diagnosis, but described the difficulties he was having tying a tie, buttoning a shirt, and walking up stairs. On a chart shown on the screen, the downturn in his batting average was compared to that of Lou Gehrig. So Frates presented the same image as Gehrig of the young athlete whose impressive physical skills were eroded by the disease. Other notable athletes have been former Yankees pitcher Jim Catfish Hunter, golfer Jeff Julian, and professional football players Glenn Montgomery and Steve Gleason. Stephen Heywood, a six-foot-two carpenter from California, the subject of Jonathan Weiner's *His Brother's Keeper*, also fits the category of the young, strong man cut down in his prime.

Another category of the public ALS patient is the **artist/performer**. In this case, the gifted artist with voice and movement loses his or her ability to walk on stage, sing or say lines, or dance. This category includes folk singer Huddie Ledbetter, as well as musicians Jason Becker, Derek Bailey, Dennis Day and Eric Lowen. Actors David Niven, Robert Webber, and Michael Zaslow fit this category. Michael Zaslow, who was a regular on the CBS soap opera "The Guiding Light," actually returned to the small screen after his diagnosis, playing a pianist stricken with ALS on ABC's "One Life to Live."

Finally, there is the **entrepreneu**r. Several of the books about ALS for a general readership portray a successful, busy person who receives the diagnosis and in a burst of energy and will—along with family and friends—organizes resources to fight the disease, to "beat this thing," and in the process displays, however briefly, those talents that had made him or her successful. Wealthy fitness guru and equipment manufacturer Augie Nieto channeled his organizational and sales skills to raise money and to help build the non-profit ALS Therapy Development Institute, dedicated to "coordinating and overseeing ALS research across the globe." Theatrical producer Jenifer Estess and her sisters similarly launched what they called Project ALS by drawing together their friends in the entertainment world—including Ben Silver, Katie Couric, and Marisa Tomei—to raise money and in the process create a "world-leading consortium."

While the possibility of triggers of ALS is still being studied, it remains a fact of the disease that all its victims are innocent. They are not the victims of their own lifestyle, eating habits, or negligence. There seems no reason at this stage to focus on preventing the disease, or in any way blaming the victim. Neurologist Stanley Appel, based on his experience at Methodist Hospital in Houston, often refers to ALS as "the nice guy's disease," citing the lack of patients who are "nervous" or "perturbed" individuals. In a very poignant way, the disease strikes innocent people sporadically and out of the blue.

The Sad Treatment History Leaving an Open Field

If a drug company is able to manufacture an effective drug or other treatment for ALS, for a while at least it will be the only hope for patients and families. There will be the exclusive rights as guaranteed by the Orphan Drug Law, but also the lack of any competition in the field, at least for a while. And the drug does not have to be a cure or a life-saver. Rilutek, the only drug currently approved for ALS, extends the life of patients only for months and actually provides no appreciable improvement in one's quality of life, yet it garners $50 million a year in proceeds from US sales and up to $300 million worldwide for its maker Aventis. Pharmaceutical firms have been started and grown based on the sales of a single original drug.

ALS researchers agree that a cure for one neurodegenerative disease may lead to a cure for another, perhaps immediately. ALS researchers such as Dr. Merit Cudkowicz are working on several diseases, such as Huntington's disease or spinal muscular atrophy, as are pharmaceutical companies such as ISIS. Often mentioned by associations and drug companies seeking a treatment for ALS is a possible connection or similarity involving ALS and Alzheimer's disease, which affects many more people than ALS and has garnered immense attention.

The Media View of the Poignant Truth

The portrait of the ALS victim, while it is rare for the average person to see it, is of someone whose body has been lost while his or her mind, senses, heart and soul are fully functioning. The heart, that involuntary muscle, keeps beating, the brain keeps wondering, and the patient continues to think and feel and act as he or she loses the ability to walk, grasp, talk, and breathe. Each patient's story, as told in local media or under the national spotlight, is compelling in that way.

Despite the millions of dollars spent annually on ALS research, the search for a cure or treatment has yielded no new therapies approved by the FDA since Rilutek in 1995. Despite the advances in our basic understanding of the genetic defects that result in ALS in FALS families, there has been no breakthrough in developing a treatment since the first gene was discovered in 1993. One of the most recent, and expensive, failures was Biogen Idec's dexpramipexole.

In announcing his company's high hopes for dexpramipexole in an April 2012 article on the business pages of *The Boston Globe*, Biogen Idec's chief executive George Scangos said, "I don't know any disease that's in more need of therapy than ALS." He was speaking both of the crying need and of the business opportunity. "It's certainly risky, but the data speaks for itself. So we made a calculated bet," he told Meg Tirrell of *Bloomberg News*. Biogen Idec paid $80 million for a licensing deal in 2010 with Knopp Biosciences, which first developed the drug, and was ready to pay an additional $265 million to Knopp if certain regulatory and sales goals were eventually met. That was the hope and the plan in April 2012 as the drug entered Phase III trials.

By January of 2013, eight months after publically expressing high hopes, the company announced that the drug had failed. News reports such as the one on the front page of *The Boston Globe* announced, "Biogen Idec's ALS Drug Falls Short in Trials." The story had both medical and financial implications. Bloomberg news was reporting by the end of the trading day that Biogen Idec's stock had dropped 1.4%, as investors' hopes, along with patients' hopes, were dashed. Biogen Idec's spokespeople, who had held out such promise just months before, were forced to put a new spin on the news. They reiterated their commitment to the search for a cure for ALS, they promised to publish the results for others to learn from, and they announced new plans and initiatives. Douglas Kerr, Biogen's director of neurodegeneration clinical research, said, "As a physician who has treated people with ALS, I hoped with all my heart for a different outcome. While these results were not what we expected, we hope these data will provide a foundation for future ALS research."

The dexpramipexole study was characterized by Rob Goldstein of the ALS Therapy Development Institute as a "really good study of what turned out to be a not-so-good drug." The Biogen Idec trial had enrolled over nine hundred patients worldwide and thereby had what scientists call "power." If the results had been positive they would have been convincing because of the size and the quality of the trial. The company and the ALS community could have hoped for quick approval by the FDA for manufacture and sales of the drug. The company itself had predicted sales of $100 million by the end of 2016, and $400 million by the end of the decade, justifying the company's investment of $80 million for the licensing rights plus the cost of the drug's trial and development.

ALS is sometimes compared to and contrasted with multiple sclerosis, both as a medical mystery and a business opportunity. In the same article in which the disappointing results of the dexpramipexole study were announced, industry analysts mentioned the company's success in marketing drugs for the treatment of MS. Biogen Idec was selling the multiple sclerosis therapies Avonex and Tysabri, and was awaiting regulatory approval of its first pill for the disease, BG-12. The new MS medicine could draw as much as $4 billion in revenue if approved, according to industry analysts as quoted in an article published in *Bloomberg News*.

In contrast to ALS patients, MS patients live longer; therefore the prevalence of the disease is larger, and the number of potential customers greater. The incidences of the two diseases—the number of new cases each year—are similar; however at any given time the number of people with MS worldwide is estimated at two-and-a-half million, whereas the number of people with ALS is estimated at only three hundred fifty thousand.

Promising Directions

At the same time that Biogen Idec and the ALS community were absorbing the meaning of the failure of dexpramipexole, research centers around the world were pursuing a large variety of other therapies and theories that could lead to new compounds for treatment. "A Cure is Coming" shouted the website of the ALS Therapy Development Institute. The science of ALS was benefiting from a number of breakthroughs in medical research in general. Researchers speak of unprecedented sharing and collaboration, and of promising projects along a number of fronts. It is not within the scope of this book to provide an exhaustive list of promising directions but to simply list a few.

Stem Cells

ALS researchers, like doctors in the centers of research for many diseases, watched with much anticipation the cloning of Dolly the ewe in Scotland in 1996, and then the growth of embryonic stem cells in the lab of University of Wisconsin scientist James Thompson in 1998. The National Academy of Science in 1995 spelled out the case:

"Because ES [embryonic stem] cells have the developmental potential to give rise to all adult cell types, any disease resulting from the failure of specific cells would be potentially treatable through the transplantation of differentiated cells derived from ES cells . . . Because of the range of diseases potentially treatable by this approach, elucidating the basic mechanism controlling the differentiation of primate ES cells has dramatic clinical significance."

In the case of ALS, for which a defective gene within cells had been identified in 1993, the promise seemed real. In her book *The Stem Cell Hope*, science writer Alice Park recounts the efforts of Jenifer Estess's group to interest doctors in stem cell pathways in 1998. Park quotes Columbia professor of biochemistry and molecular biophysics Thomas Jessell applying stem cell theory to ALS and other neurodegenerative diseases. "If one understands at a fundamental level the way a neural circuit assembles itself for function, then you have a better chance of intervening and manipulating that circuit under conditions when things start to go wrong," Jessell explained.

In April of 2013, the FDA approved Phase II of a clinical trial of stem cell therapy for ALS patients to be led by University of Michigan neurologist Dr. Eva Feldman. Fifteen patients had been part of the Phase I tolerability study, conducted at Emory University. One of those patients was Ted Harada whose story was mentioned in Chapter 8. In Phase II, at both Emory and the University of Michigan, Dr. Feldman and colleagues would be overseeing the injection of up to four hundred thousand stem cells per injection into the upper part of the spinal cord of ALS patients, and monitoring safety and tolerability, as well as the effect on the patients' disease progression.

Gene Therapy

The idea behind gene therapy is to transplant genes into cells, effectively rewriting their DNA. It is gene transplantation, using a vector or delivery vehicle, such as a virus, to safely carry a working version of the gene into the cell. In 1999, however, the promise of gene therapy was dashed with the death of Jesse Gelsinger, a Pennsylvania teenager, in a clinical trial in Philadelphia. In Jesse's case, the good copies of genes were inserted into the patient within a virus. Shortly after being injected with the virus, Gelsinger's temperature rose dramatically and soon the young man's body was seized with inflammation. He was taken off life support days later. The particular researchers in this case were criticized by the FDA for making several critical mistakes, and with failing to inform Jesse and his parents of prior problems with humans in the trial. The momentum for this form of therapy was lost for a time.

In recent years, according to *The Boston Globe*, gene therapy has rebounded as methods have been found to increase the safety of the procedure. An article in *Wired* magazine in September of 2013 reported on the career of James Wilson, formerly the director of the University of Pennsylvania's Institute for Human Gene Therapy—the same institute that had treated Jesse Gelsinger. After Gelsinger's death, his career almost ruined, Wilson stayed in the field to learn of the errors made and to find a way to deliver the promise of gene therapy more safely.

In February of 2014, a new Boston biotech startup, Voyager Therapeutics, announced its plans to use a class of viruses known as adeno-associated viruses as carriers to deliver vital proteins to the brain. The company will target Parkinson's Disease and ALS. On its website the company described its plans for correcting the SOD1 protein, writing, "By knocking down SOD1, our goal is to reduce the level of mutated SOD1 protein in the CNS [central nervous system] and have a meaningful impact on the progression of the disease."

The promise of stem cells and gene therapy, then, is the promise of replacement or transplantation, to replace the bad cells and bad genes with good ones. In *The Boston Globe* article, Dr. Robert Brown is quoted as saying that the promise of the technique for ALS researchers and families is in the possibility that toxic genes could be "silenced." His colleague Craig Mello won the Nobel Prize for medicine in 2006 for his work in showing how malfunctioning genes could be shut down.

ISIS Pharmaceuticals and Antisense Therapy

At the same time that Biogen Idec was announcing the negative trial results of its drug dexpramipexole, ISIS Pharmaceuticals and its research sites were publishing the results of the Phase I trial of what they were then calling ISIS 333611, the therapeutic approach that had been touted with much hope by Dr. Merit Cudkowicz in talking with Mary Prior and her siblings in January of 2010.

Antisense technology, as described in Chapter 8 when it was first introduced to Mary Prior, operates at the level of ribonucleic acid or RNA, a polymeric molecule implicated in various biological roles in coding, decoding, regulation, and expression of genes. As the company's website explains it, antisense technology promises "a direct route from genomics to drugs." The antisense strand is one of the two sides of that familiar twisted ladder-like image of DNA. The nucleotides on one side of the ladder interact with nucleotides on the other side across the steps of the ladder. Scientists at ISIS have been studying ways to create drugs that bind to nucleotides to interrupt the process of producing the toxic protein. For ALS patients, it is designed to block production of the toxic protein that is found in people with the SOD1 gene mutation. The ISIS trial was described as a "watershed moment" by R. Rodney Howell, a metabolic disease specialist and chairman of the MDA Board of Directors.

In the March 2013 article in the journal *Lancet Neurology*, Dr. Timothy Miller and his colleagues at six sites, including Dr. Cudkowicz at Mass General, summarized their findings from Phase I of the trial. The drug had proven to be safe and tolerable when given to twenty one individuals with FALS using the intrathecal delivery method injecting it directly into the spinal fluid of the subjects. Nine of the participants received multiple doses by re-enrolling in subsequent cohorts, eight—two in each cohort—received a placebo. Four dose levels were evaluated sequentially. The study also evaluated the pharmacokinetics of the drug and the delivery method; that is, the successful distribution of the drug in people.

The intrathecal delivery method had proven tolerable, even though it was a twelve hour procedure, and in some cases resulted in the kinds of headaches that patients get when they receive an epidural anesthetic or undergo a spinal tap. The brief *Lancet* article reported side effects including post-lumbar puncture syndrome, back pain and nausea. But, they reported, "We recorded no dose-limiting toxic effects or any safety or tolerability concerns related to ISIS 333611. No serious adverse events occurred in patients given ISIS 333611." In addition, "Re-enrollment and re-treatment were also well tolerated," the authors reported.

Interviewed in April of 2013, Dr. Cudkowicz of MGH and Dr. Frank Bennett, senior Vice President of Research at ISIS, provided a summary of the trial and their plans for the future. According to Dr. Bennett, while the ISIS Phase I trial was in progress, he and his colleagues at ISIS had been conducting more nonhuman toxicology tests, and had learned a lot more about the drug and its potential. This new knowledge allowed them to create a slightly different compound that may have wider applications to FALS. Their plan was to eventually submit this new compound for FDA approval with the hope that the FDA's confidence born from the first trial would allow it to approve the new compound quickly for a clinical trial, and to accelerate the trial process. The new trial of the ISIS antisense compound might also allow for multiple doses and for sick FALS patients to join the trial in Phase I and then receive potentially effective doses in Phase II.

The brief and tentative message of hope first given to Mary Prior and her family in January of 2010 might soon be extended to other patients and their families. Dr. Bennett, in discussing the ISIS history, confirmed that contributions of the Farrs and other families at several stages had been instrumental in bringing his firm to this science. The Farrs had contributed to Dr. Brown's work, which had in turn, Bennett said, "created opportunities for firms to examine genetic pathways and to find compounds to interrupt those diseased pathways or to restore the good ones." In addition, he acknowledged, Susan Lynaugh's advocacy for research and trial participants in a webinar had helped the sites recruit a few more FALS patients to the trial after a slow start. ISIS Pharmaceuticals was planning a brief hiatus to study the new antisense oligonucle-otide compound before reapplying to the FDA. As this book went to press, ISIS had announced no new trial of the new compound in ALS patients.

In the meantime, according to Dr. Cudkowicz, her colleague Dr. Timothy Miller is studying ways to measure the levels of SOD1 in ALS patients, and even in FALS family members at risk for the disease. Someday, therefore, antisense therapy may even have a preventive potential, lowering the levels of the toxic protein in people so that they never develop symptoms. The news in the spring of 2013 allowed the family to keep the hope alive that, as Dr. Cudkowicz had said to Mary Prior, future generations of Farrs may not have to go through what their brothers, sisters, aunts and uncles, as well as their distant ancestors had gone through.

Affecting Immune Cells

Several ALS researchers and pharmaceutical companies are studying ways to affect the immune system by blocking, suppressing, or transforming immune cells.

The ALS Therapy Development Institute in Cambridge, MA is a unique nonprofit organization devoted to surveying the full landscape of activity to find a cure for ALS. Its mission is to evaluate potential therapies wherever they may emerge and in whatever setting. Launched in 1999 by Jamie Heywood months after his brother Stephen was diagnosed with ALS, ALS TDI sees itself as the world's first nonprofit biotech institute. Today it has grown to be an "industrial scale," preclinical evaluator of potential therapeutics. The institute employs thirty professional scientists and operates a large, state-of – the-art, fifteen-thousand square foot laboratory at its Kendall Square address in the heart of Cambridge's academic and biotech neighborhood.

Until recently, ALS TDI was not involved in clinical trials. ALS TDI researchers would study a particular set of ideas, as basic science, then take those ideas as far as the creation of a compound to test on mice. The institute sought partners to conduct trials on humans. At various stages in its drug development program, ALS TDI has partnered with universities, MDA and ALS associations, large and small pharmaceutical firms, and private foundations. Rob Goldstein of ALS TDI refers to the institute's methodology as "venture philanthropy." The institute does acquire some intellectual property rights in the process of its investigations and may at a later date sell or financially benefit from those assets. All funds, however, remain with the nonprofit. In February of 2013, in a new development, ALS TDI announced that it had received FDA approval to conduct its own clinical trials in ALS patients.

The drug to be tested was actually a drug manufactured and sold by the large pharmaceutical firm Novartis for treatment of multiple sclerosis. The drug is fingolimod, marketed as Gilenya, and was first approved for MS in 2010. The FDA approved a trial for ALS starting in Phase IIA, meaning that its main purpose was still to test for safety and tolerability in ALS patients, but since the drug was already being taken by thousands of MS patients, ALS TDI can start ALS patients on larger doses and test for the appropriate dosage. Phase IIB follows, in which the efficacy of the drug is monitored to see if it is actually affecting symptoms.

As described in the press release when the trial was announced, Gilenya works by blocking "certain immune cells from entering the brain and spinal cord where they can cause activities that result in damage to motor neurons." As described by Novartis, "The immune system contains a network of lymph nodes, which are tiny glands containing immune cells called lymphocytes. Lymphocytes are normally good guys, but sometimes they can go rogue. This can mean they go after your central nervous system and cause problems. While it's not exactly clear how Gilenya works, it is thought to keep lymphocytes from attacking your central nervous system by lowering the number of lymphocytes circulating in your blood." ALS TDI's own preclinical studies of the compound, which it is calling TSI-132, had determined that it significantly reduced the circulation of the immune cells through the blood stream of mice.

Another therapy that may affect immune cells is Neuraltus's NP001, which aims to transform macrophages, a type of immune cell, from an activated, neurotoxic, inflammatory state to a neuroprotective state. The immune-suppression regimen including prednisone mentioned in Chapter 8, the trial in which Clif

Langmaid was enrolled, is another therapy being tested.

Protein Misfolding

While ALS researchers in many medical centers are searching for toxic substances in cells, for rogue chemical reactions, and viruses, others are looking at a simple bio-mechanical process gone wrong. It is called protein folding. Scientists studying this pathway speak in physical terms of folding, unfolding and misfolding, funnels, cells, chains, structural components, three dimensional structures, original native forms and configurations, even nooks and crannies. As scientist Enrique Reynaud explains it, "Proteins fold into their minimal-energy configuration because of the physicochemical properties of their amino acid sequence. Proteins fold rapidly because amino acids interact locally, thus limiting the conformational space that the protein has to explore and forcing the protein to follow a funnel-like landscape that allows it to fold quickly."

Proteins are essential for proper cell function, and the proper folding of the proteins into the correct shape is essential for their normal function. Reynaud compares DNA and the genome to a tightly packed digital MP3 file which contains the information to make proteins. When something goes wrong, the protein folds into a very different structure than its native one. It is said to misfold.

The explorations of Amorfix Life Sciences, a Canadian company, are based on these findings about what they call Aggregated Misfolded Proteins, or AMPs. The company is developing both therapeutic products, which may be able to fix or neutralize the effects of these misfolded protein structures, and diagnostic products, which may be able to detect them and in the process diagnose ALS.

Neurite Outgrowth Inhibition

Studies with monkeys, SOD1 mice, and ALS patients, have suggested to scientists that a protein called NOGO-A is a possible inhibitor of neuron growth in ALS patients. The neurons are the primary motor pathways connecting the central nervous system and muscles. The death of these neurons leads to the muscular effects—spasticity, shrinking, and hyper-reflexia—that debilitate ALS patients. The NOGO-A protein is not found in healthy muscle tissue but is prevalent in the skeletal muscle tissue of ALS patients and victims. The protein also seems to disrupt the normal process at the neuromuscular junction, where the neuron connects to the muscle.

The goal in synthesizing a NOGO-A antibody, then, is to administer a chemical that "neutralizes or antagonizes" the growth of a protein which inhibits the growth of neurons. The antibody currently in clinical trials is GlaxoSmith Kline's GSK1223249. Their trial began in 2009. As of May 2013, the trial had moved into Phase II after finding no adverse effects in Phase I.

GlaxoSmithKline is also recommending the expression of NOGO-A as a diagnostic biomarker. A study of thirty-three patients with problems in lower motor function found NOGO-A in seventeen but not in the other sixteen. However, within twelve months a follow-up study found that ninety-one percent of those patients who were later diagnosed with ALS did have the NOGO-A protein in their biopsy samples, so a test of people starting to have trouble with muscle weakening could lead to a prediction that, yes, it is going to develop into ALS.

Neuron and Axon Vulnerability

While scientists and pharmaceutical companies continue the ever-more-widening search for the molecular and genetic pathways of ALS, the focus on the actual mechanical junctions has not disappeared. It is known, for instance, that in ALS patients the axon, the tip of the neuron where it connects to the muscle, retracts. The synaptic gap widens. The Swiss biotech company Neurotone, which has specialized in developing medicines for neuropathic pain and for age related loss of muscle strength, is working with the ALS Therapy Development Institute to develop a compound that may improve—or forestall the loss of—strength, connectivity, and stability of neurons at the juncture.

Muscle Contractility and Bulbar Control

A heart medicine named mexiletine is being tested to see if it can reduce the hyper-excitability of muscles that lead to cramping. In this case an FDA-approved drug for one purpose—regulating heart rhythm—is being retested for a use in another type of patient. If it works, mexiletine may reduce discomfort, and perhaps slow the progress of the disease by reducing the over-activity of sodium channels on certain neurons.

The drug company Cytokinetics has developed medicines to help muscles contract more smoothly by affecting the sarcomere, the fundamental unit of skeletal muscle contraction. Cytokinetics refers to its drug CK-2017357 as a "fast skeletal muscle troponin activator," which increases the muscle's sensitivity to calcium.

ALS and Dementia

As stated many times in this book, ALS robs the patient of his or her body but seems to leave the mind functioning well. It may even sharpen the mind, as the philosopher-patients have testified. However, not always. Some patients, including Farrs, have seemed to become more forgetful and less sharp in the years leading up to their development of ALS.

In an April 2013 article in the journal *Neuroscience* entitled "The Changing Scene of Amyotrophic Lateral Sclerosis," authors Wim Robberecht of Belgium and Thomas Phillips of Johns Hopkins summarized the current thinking about the disease worldwide. On the subject of dementia, they wrote, "breakthroughs have revealed mechanistic links between ALS and frontotemporal dementia [FTLD]." There is such a thing as ALS-FTLD, which, according to Robberecht and Phillips, affects fifteen percent of all ALS patients. "This suggests," they write, "that ALS and FTLD are two ends of the spectrum of one disease." Also on that spectrum, are ALS with cognitive or behavioral impairment (ALS-Ci/Bi), and fronto-temporal dementia with mild motor neuron involvement

(FTLD-MND). The concept of the spectrum was confirmed by the discovery in 2011 of a particular chromosome mutation (C9orf72) as a common cause for both ALS and FTLD.

The mystery of why the age of onset of ALS varies so widely has only deepened with recent discoveries. The connection between ALS and FTLD suggests that both are functions of aging, but why did Curtis Vance get sick at age twenty-five, his grandmother at forty, his aunt Mary at sixty-three, and his great-grandmother at seventy-nine? As the authors put the question, "Why do mutant proteins that are present from the beginning of an individual's life only cause a disease after several decades, which is then fatal within a couple of years?" That is the other half of the question, then: not only why does age of onset vary, but why then does the disease progress so quickly?

Environmental Triggers

The question *What triggers ALS* is still a very live issue, according to Dr. Elijah Stommel of Dartmouth Hitchcock Medical Center, interviewed early in 2014. It is of interest to both sporadic ALS sufferers and their families, and to FALS families. For an apparently sporadic case, especially an early onset case, the question is: what was I exposed to that might have "caused" ALS? As mentioned earlier, suspects have included pesticides, heavy metals, fish and other elements of diet, and pond scum. In several of these hypotheses, a common denominator was amino acids, the BMAA referred to in the section on Guam in Chapter 3. The NFL Players Association wants to know the reason for the prevalence of ALS among former players. With concentrated attention being given to head trauma in the NFL, researchers noticed a higher incidence of ALS among players in the speed positions, as opposed to linemen. The Pentagon has studied the higher incidence of ALS among Gulf War veterans. Of particular interest to scientists like Dr. Stommel are the rare but real cases of spouses who both came down with the symptoms of sporadic ALS. In those cases, you would have to assume that the cause is environmental.

For a FALS family, there is an awareness that, although they have a genetic disposition toward ALS, nevertheless there are mysterious patterns of early onset, late onset and no onset—the obligate carriers who never got sick. It is natural for the family to wonder about triggers; they may give them a kind of hope, especially in the face of a positive genetic test or parental history, that even though they have the toxic gene, something still has to set it off, and maybe that something can be avoided.

In its basic progress once diagnosed, amyotrophic lateral sclerosis is a homogeneous disorder, especially for a family that has seen a number of cases. Aspects of the disease may vary (such as age of onset), but essentially, it is going to progressively move around the body weakening virtually all muscle groups. In its basic symptoms, FALS, whether resulting from the SOD1 gene defect or another genetic cause, progresses and shows itself identically to the sporadic forms of the disease. It is said to be "clinically similar." This fact, in the family consciousness, explains why there was a natural expectation that the disease would someday be understood as having a single cause. And when the SOD1 gene was isolated in 1993, the family as well as many in the medical field and in the general public felt that *the cause* had been found. Farr family members still talk that way: the cause has been found.

"However, ALS turns out to be a very heterogeneous disorder," wrote Robberecht and Phillips in the spring of 2013. Mutations in the SOD1 gene, over a hundred, can result in a variety of phenotypes, including classic ALS, progressive muscular atrophy, frontotemporal dementia, parkinsonism, and even psychosis. Since 1993 and the discovery of the SOD1 gene defect, over thirty more genetic causes have been found. The complexity of the disease increases with every new probing of the cause or causes.

In an essay entitled "Controversies and Priorities in Amyotrophic Lateral Sclerosis," published in the journal *Lancet Neurology* in March of 2013, which was written as a summary of the issues discussed at an ALS conference in Sydney, Australia in the fall of 2012, authors Martin R. Turner and Matthew Kiernan, writing on behalf of twenty contributors, ask several basic, penetrating questions about the way we have viewed ALS since Charcot:

- Has the concept of ALS as one disease become untenable?

- Can apparently sporadic ALS be inherited?

- Is physical activity itself, being very fit and thin, actually "harmful to a minority of the population who carry a complex genetic profile?"

The authors of the "Controversies" article base their questions on the increasing awareness of the genetic diversity among ALS patients, sporadic and familial, and to the "monumental discovery" in 2011 that "a substantial proportion of the remainder of cases of FALS [non-SOD1 families] have now been traced to an expansion of the intronic hexanucleotide repeat sequence in C9orf72."

C9orf72 Gains the Spotlight

Between 1993 and 2011, the focus of Dr. Robert Brown and other researchers had been on understanding all cases of ALS by trying to understand the cause of the disease in SOD1 families. That all began to shift, however, with the discovery of this new genetic abnormality—C9orf72. The significant difference between SOD1 and C9orf72 is in the fact that the C9orf72 defect has also been linked to fronto-temporal dementia (FTD) and has been found in cases of sporadic ALS. Studies at the Mayo Clinic found the genetic changes in twelve percent of cases of FTD and twenty-three percent of cases of familial ALS, in three percent of cases of sporadic FTD, and four percent of cases of sporadic ALS. The C9orf72 defect as a genetic cause of FALS was particularly prevalent in Europe; one study co-authored by Dr. Brown and fourteen colleagues around the world found the C9orf72 defect to be present in various countries in proportions ranging from twenty to eighty-six percent of the cases not previously diagnosed as familial cases of FALS/FTD.

In these cases of the C9orf72 abnormality, researchers found that "a short DNA sequence is repeated many more times as compared to healthy individuals," as explained in an ALS Association bulletin. The expanded repeat section may bind tightly to certain proteins, forming "clumps" within the brain cells which may prevent the proteins from carrying out their normal functions in the cell. Researchers immediately set out to create a mouse model for C9orf72, and to research forms of possible treatment.

The SOD1 gene defect remains an important focus of study, however, because this FALS population is still quite large, much has been invested in understanding the disease mechanism, and the mouse models are still very useful. In addition, in October of 2013, Amorfix Life Sciences announced that it had found the presence of misfolded SOD1 in sporadic cases of ALS. Calling SOD1 the "Jekyll and Hyde protein," due to its function as a positive anti-oxidant in its native configuration but harmful in its altered state, Amorfix pledged to continue its efforts to find a therapeutic treatment for SOD1 FALS, possibly as a vaccine, and also a diagnostic test based on its ability to identify misfolded SOD1 in presymptomatic subjects.

Precision Medicine

During his January 2015 State of the Union Address, President Barack Obama made brief mention of the White House initiative which he called Precision Medicine. He said, "I want the country that eliminated polio and mapped the human genome to lead a new era of medicine—one that delivers the right treatment at the right time. In some patients with cystic fibrosis, this approach has reversed a disease once thought unstoppable. Tonight, I am launching a new Precision Medicine Initiative to bring us closer to curing diseases like cancer and diabetes—and to give all of us access to personalized information we need to keep ourselves and our families healthier." The White House pledged $215 million to the initiative.

In follow-up, the ALS Therapy Development Institute defined precision medicine as "a field which aims to leverage genomic data together with an individual's own medical history and disease symptoms and progression to more rapidly identify potential therapies." ALS TDI's own program, launched in 2013, plans to enroll hundreds of patients living with ALS—familial or sporadic—and pledged to fully sequence each patient's genome, keep track of each patient's symptoms through self-reporting and clinical testing, create an induced pluripotent stem cell line from each patient's biopsy, and to use those stem cell lines to study mechanisms of the disease and search for possible treatments. The institute also pledged to share all data with the participants. In April of 2015, ALS TDI announced the enrollment of its hundredth patient, with hundreds more waiting to be screened.

· · · · ·

To patients and families, the lack of a cure or effective treatment, coupled with the discoveries that the disease may be even more complex and variable than previously thought, may be discouraging. There will be no magic bullet, no breakthrough leading immediately to *a cure*. Not only is the cause of the disease going to turn out to be "multifactorial," but, it seems, so are the causes of the causes. Muscle loss results from synaptic dysfunction and axonal withdrawal right where the axon brings signals to the muscle, but even the mechanism affecting that process "appears multifactorial." And don't tell a family that has suffered from progressive muscle atrophy for over 150 years that the concept of ALS as one disease is untenable.

To scientists and neurologists, however, looking at the long history of this disease, all of the recent discoveries, and all of the current theories, therapies, and trials mean progress. Progress in getting to a basic understanding of the disease will lead to a cure or treatment. The history of research into ALS and other diseases tells us that shots in the dark rarely hit the target. Quackery and patent medicines, few-patient trials without controls, or small and short trials, and solitary scientists in their labs have rarely ever led to anything. While there is still a lively debate within the profession about what constitutes a good enough clinical trial, and what is a reliable indicator or bio-marker and what is a false positive, leading researchers call for patience and continuing hard work without taking shortcuts. Today, thanks to modern attitudes and the internet, ALS researchers communicate, share and collaborate. "Progress in our understanding of the mechanism underlying ALS over the past decade has been substantial," write Robberecht and Phillips. "The more complex, the more opportunity." The authors of the "Controversies" essay also point to some unity within the diversity of current opinions. There is a "unifying pathogenic theme of nuclear protein mishandling in ALS," they write, a fact which they call "tantalizing."

What is likely to happen in the search for a cure for ALS is that not one magic bullet or single vaccine but multiple treatments will be used to target the many forms of the disease which result from different mutated genes. To Dr. Robert Brown himself, there has been real progress in getting a clear "sense of the cause," of ALS. As he described it in the summer of 2013, we are now looking through the "molecular keyhole" of the doorway to a cure, and although there is much work to be done, at least we are knocking on the right door. In particular, there is realistic hope for patients and families with a certain genetic makeup that a cure or treatment will be found to turn off, reprogram, compensate for, or circumnavigate the pathway of that particular toxic gene. The Farrs and other SOD1 families are still among the most likely candidates to first receive that benefit and relief.

Dr. Robert H. Brown Jr. has stated, "It is possible that the first types of ALS to be treated will be those that have been so devastating to this wonderful family."

To Be A FALS Family

W ithin the ALS community, there is an abbreviation for patients with ALS (PALS), for sporadic cases of ALS (SALS), and for families with a history of ALS (FALS). Families of sporadic victims when a family member gets sick may tend to make a very quick study of the disease, and then after the loss of their loved one, resume their lives with the knowledge that it will probably not strike again. It is a rare disease. However, they remain sympathetic and may remain active in fundraising and the search for a cure.

To be a FALS member is to be more aware of one's own family history as well as the history of the disease. I have found a large spectrum among Farr family members in what they know, and how often they think, about the disease, but a FALS member knows the science, or knows someone in the family who is up on the science. According to doctors and others in the field, most FALS families are known by a single name, such as the Farrs, to simplify things, as well as a number in the lab, and by their gene if it is known. When Curtis Vance got sick and tried to get an appointment at a major medical center, his mother told him, "Tell them you're a Farr." At first it didn't work; the name meant nothing to the appointment scheduler at Dartmouth Hitchcock Medical Center. At Massachusetts General Hospital's ALS Clinic, however, it worked; Curtis got an immediate appointment. Dr. Merit Cudkowicz of MGH has treated four members of the Vermont Farr family.

To be a FALS family, then, is to receive special treatment. At Massachusetts General Hospital, they know the family history and the fact that the family's particular mutation of the SOD1 gene is the A4V, fast-progressing type; there isn't a lot of time. With the increasing focus on genetics in the understanding of ALS, there will be a different treatment for each genetic mutation, and to have a prominent and widespread mutation in a gene such as SOD1 or C9orf72 may mean that treatments for it will come first. Because the function of the normal gene is better understood, the faulty mechanism of the defective gene is better understood, and treatments may be developed to correct it or to compensate for it. The antisense therapies of ISIS Pharmaceuticals, for instance, are gene-specific.

To be a FALS family, however, is to remember and forget. Family members live with the knowledge of the family history, and of others' first symptoms, while trying to put it all out of their minds to live their daily lives. They are not deniers, but they find ways to avoid thinking about it daily. Some of my sources, who not coincidentally are on a "safe" branch of the family without a victim among their parents, have surprisingly little knowledge of the disease, or the family history, and think about it rarely. Some of the family members who have been my best sources for this book, on the other hand, say they are not sure they will be able to read it, because it will be too real and painful. A new member of the family gets sick and one reaction is, "I am just so tired of losing my loved ones." It may even account for the fact that they are not in close touch with cousins who live out of the area.

Most members of a FALS family, however, do notice the latest developments in understanding of, or treatment for, the disease, and hope springs inevitably. They know about clinical trials, and may even check the NIH's website clinicaltrials.gov for a posting of the latest ALS trial. There were 743 clinical trials that listed ALS in early 2015. Fifty-eight were listed for Massachusetts General Hospital, either in the recruiting phase, active and not recruiting, or recently completed or abandoned. FALS families may naturally place their hopes on a particular trial at a nearby site. They also tend to place their faith in certain doctors and researchers.

To be an FALS family activist, however, is to be rankled by several of the realities of medicine today and by ALS's orphan status. Associated as they are with one disease, and having suffered as a family for over 150 years, family activists are understandably impatient with the slow progress of science; they can't understand why after all these years there is no cure or treatment. Who are "compassionate doses" for if not for a FALS patient? Where are the investors and the big donors? The attention given to other diseases—the fundraisers, the developments trumpeted on the evening news, the endless advertisements encouraging you to "Ask your doctor about" the latest medicine, the official sponsors and the community-wide rallies, walks, and "wars"—is a constant source of irritation and envy to a FALS family. That changed at least temporarily during the summer of 2014 with the Ice Bucket Challenge, which resulted in an amazing infusion of funds, and attention and awareness, to the family disease. Still, when everyone is wearing pink at a nationally televised sporting event, it is hard to watch. Meanwhile, ALS is the official charity of minor league baseball.

Patient guides provide excellent advice for caregivers. *Amyotrophic Lateral Sclerosis: A Guide for Patients and Families* contains a five-chapter section on living with the reality of ALS, with essays on support groups, meditation, family caregivers, financial realities, and home care agencies. The diagnosis of ALS for the patient and family, the guide says, is a "life-changing event. One's sense of self is threatened, and one cannot help but question why this has occurred." We can only imagine what it is like for a member of a FALS family to go through the whole, sad experience nine times in a lifetime. It seems to result in a form of battle fatigue, of great weariness, to summon the energy to care once again, and to rekindle some small ember of hope.

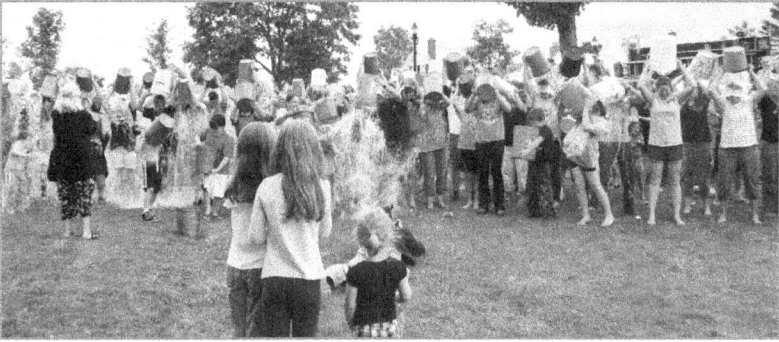

The Ice Bucket Challenge—Danville Green September 21, 2014.

CHAPTER 10

The Next Generation

"When my aunt came down with the disease she called me aside and told me never to have children because I would not want them to get this disease through me now would I? However, I decided that there are a lot of diseases and things that can happen to people so I would go ahead and have my family as I had planned, and if anyone would get this I was sure it would only be me anyway, and I could handle it for myself."

Linda Vance, in her letter to her son

Every descendent of Erastus Farr has a decision to make, or rather many decisions. There are odds here to be calculated, awful and hopeful scenarios to play out in his or her mind, and a certain amount of soul-searching depending on self-knowledge. How important are children to me? How long will I myself live? My husband does not have the gene; will he outlive me, and what will he want for that part of his life? What are my other health risk factors; what else might end my life before I get ALS, if I get ALS?

Should I get tested? What evidence is there that my mother, my father, or I have the defective gene? Is there anything I can change in my lifestyle to make it less likely that I'll get ALS?

If a young woman knows, as Linda Vance did in 1964, that her mother had the SOD1 gene defect and died of ALS, then she knows that she has a 50/50 chance of carrying the defective gene herself. If she has the defective gene, she has a high probability of developing symptoms herself. But when? At what age? What will trigger the onset of symptoms? Will there be a method of treatment or cure when she gets ALS? If that same woman sees her son develop symptoms, then she knows that she too has the defective gene, passed on to her from her mother and passed on from her to her son. By the same token, if she has seen her aunts and cousins die of the disease but watched her mother or father—whoever is in the family line—grow into old age and die leaving healthy children, then she can go to sleep at night with only a tiny flicker of worry.

If you are a Farr, there are essentially two ways of establishing a genetic cause of ALS in your immediate family: by looking at the family tree, or by being tested. All Farrs know that they are an SOD1 family, that ancestors have died from ALS, and that the defective family gene is SOD1. Some members of the Farr family know a lot more about the science than others, but all are aware at some level that there is a genetic cause. Looking at the family tree, however, the picture can be confusing, because the patterns of illness within the Vermont family, plus the Georgia contingent, are as varied and seemingly unpredictable as in the general population. It is like flipping a coin: you have a 50-50 chance of getting heads, but you may get eight tails in a row.

It can look, for instance, like women are the carriers. From Tennie's mother, Mary Matilda, to Tennie to her daughter Clara to her daughter Linda that seems to have been a pattern. Since Mary Matilda's death in 1919, no one in the Vermont branches of the family has developed ALS after having received the defective gene from his or her dad. But that is not the case historically, nor is it the science. There are other patterns within the family. Each of the known carriers of the disease who lived a long life and died of other causes was a woman.

For the Danville Farrs, from 1966 to 1988, it looked to members of the family like ALS "skipped a generation," but that was denying that Grammy Tennie died of ALS. Then came news of Kelly Ralston in 1988, and then Curtis in 1998. Counting Grammy Tennie, then, it affected every generation.

Age of onset seemed to follow the textbook norms. Six of eight family members who developed ALS did so between the ages of forty and sixty-nine. But then there was Tennie who died at seventy-nine, Rena Longchamps at seventy, and Curtis, who died at twenty-six.

In addition to studying the family tree, in the modern era, there is the possibility of genetic testing, which is preceded and followed by genetic counseling. Through testing, members of a family can find out whether any are carrying the defective gene. But do they want to know? Even if someone tests positive for the gene mutation, that does not mean that he or she has or will get the disease. It does mean that she or he is likely to; ninety percent of all SOD1 family members (those who have tested positive for the gene defect) will begin to show symptoms by age seventy. The knowledge, positive or negative, that results from testing affects the whole family. A positive test reveals that a family member is either A) already affected by changes in the body's function but not recognizing symptoms yet, B) a future victim who will one day show the outward symptoms, or C) a carrier who may be in the ten percent who live into old age without symptoms. In the Vermont/Georgia Farr family, it has happened twice since 1988 that a man in his fifties developed symptoms of ALS after his mother died without ever showing symptoms. Two mothers have seen a child diagnosed with ALS, thereby having to face the fact that they are carriers of the defective gene.

A negative test for the gene defect may help a family relax and go on with their lives with the knowledge that the person tested is not going to develop symptoms of the disease and is not going to pass on the gene to his or her offspring. It also relieves his or her parent of guilt. However, there is such a thing in FALS families as survivor's guilt. Watching a parent, sibling, cousin, niece or nephew suffer from the disease, knowing that you are not going to get it can bring on profound feelings of "Why not me?" Linda Vance firmly believes that her grandmother Tennie did not have ALS but wanted to, feeling that it was her fate, perhaps even her just penalty, for having passed on the gene to her daughters.

If a person tests positive, it is still possible that she will never have symptoms before she dies of something else, but her children will live with the knowledge that their mother was a carrier. It works in reverse, too. Suppose a mother in her forties does not want to be tested but her twenty-year old son does. If the son tests positive for the gene defect, that knowledge affects everyone in the family, and in particular it tells his mother that she has the gene and is right at the most common age of onset—a very difficult fact to live with. For this reason, FALS researchers, such as Diane McKenna-Yasek at the University of Massachusetts Medical School do much counseling before and after testing. Members of the family have told me that they were discouraged from being tested—or from finding out the results—by medical authorities for just that reason, and because there is no cure, and because it might affect their insurance coverage.

Of the eighty-four children, grandchildren and great grand-children of Tennie Toussaint, to my knowledge no one has chosen to be tested for the SOD1 gene and then opted to learn the results. Several have donated blood for testing for the benefit of medical science without wanting to know the results. One family was understood by others to have been tested but the father of the family told me he "chickened out." He did, however, save his children's umbilical cord blood, frozen for possible later testing. I have interviewed two members of the wider Farr family—not descendants of Tennie—who have been tested and learned the results. Both were on what we might call "safe" branches of the family, with no known immediate ancestors with the disease. Both tested negative.

Imagine a young woman of the Farr family, recently married, and contemplating having children. She has seen her mother die from the disease in her forties and knows at least some of the family history. The disease from her vantage point seems to affect women and not until they are in their forties, so she may reason that, if she has children, she could enjoy them for at least twenty years before they would lose her, or for forty or fifty years before she could lose them, and maybe they themselves would not get sick and live on happily after she was gone. A young mother could reason that way, and if her maternal instinct is strong she could not stop herself from having children and hoping for the best.

In addition, a gene-carrier may know that some members of the family before him or her had carried the defective gene but never got sick. You supposedly have a ninety percent chance of getting the disease, but maybe not until you are ninety-five. Tennie Toussaint died at age seventy-nine of either ALS or a stroke. Her daughter Rena, after surviving several bouts of cancer, perhaps died of ALS at age seventy. Tennie's daughter Viola Ralston lived to be eighty-five and never developed symptoms; however, she lived long enough to see her son Kelly die of ALS at age forty-three.

Suppose heart disease or some other ailment runs in the family, too. Forrest Langmaid, Linda's father, had his first heart attack at fifty-seven. His brother Arnold had his first heart attack at fifty-four. Forrest was not in the genetic line to inherit the FALS gene, but his children are all in the line to inherit what looks like genetic heart disease. Linda's brother Clif suffered a massive heart attack requiring quadruple bypass heart surgery at fifty-seven, the same age as his father, something he had always dreaded. As Linda wrote, there are a lot of diseases and things that can happen. Other health problems that run in the family are diabetes, cancer, and obesity. There is solid logic to every decision and enough permutations and combinations in life that a Farr descendent might reasonably decide to marry or not, to have children or not, to watch his or her weight or cholesterol or blood pressure or not, to live life with extreme caution—or live it with abandon.

Diane McKenna-Yasek of the University of Massachusetts, in a symposium for FALS families, referred to what she called "the deniers." Researchers like her would like to bring the deniers into the fold of what she calls "the activists." However, deniers, she acknowledged, "have a very useful defense mechanism." There is no benefit to them or to the family around them to be judgmental or to attempt to "break through" their denial. They may wish to distance themselves from the family, and that is their right. Who is to judge? Many FALS families exhibit the two poles of activism and withdrawal, with many in between.

In my research I have not met anyone in the Farr family who denies the science and reality of FALS, but I have encountered different reactions to that reality. One reaction may be to decide not to have children, as Linda Vance's aunt advised her. In Linda's mother's generation, all of Clara's brothers and sisters had children. In Linda's generation, her brother Clif never married, and her sister Jane has not married or had children. Of Linda's nieces and nephews, most have married and had children, but a few have not, or at least not yet. Of course, I do not know all the reasons.

The common in-between attitude is one of avoiding the subject within the family (although not so easy a thing to do in the mind). Just don't talk about it, don't become a student of the disease, don't sit your children down and have "the talk," don't get tested, don't become an activist. Enjoy your life and family and bond with them on all sorts of other subjects and experiences, but not ALS. Don't become obsessed. As Kim Prior, Mary and Hollis Prior's daughter, put it, "There is obsession and there is life!" The large Vance family, for instance, enjoys ocean cruises, all-terrain vehicles, hunting, little league baseball, and all sorts of family endeavors. They talk more about those interests than about ALS. When the disease strikes a member of the family, especially if the victim is living in Vermont, it brings the family history back to mind every day and the family rallies to help.

Among those families whom I have had the privilege of knowing and who have opened up their lives and relationships to me, I have noted some separation among cousins, nieces and nephews. In quite a few cases, the reasons are those common in all families. In several cases, for instance, the distance seems geographical or even cultural—they live at some distance from each other, they just don't see each other much, and they don't seem to have much in common. Work, such as farming, keeps you close to home. In some cases, the estrangement seems to be caused by other common factors: a messy divorce, sibling rivalry, jealousy, or some past slight or injury. In other cases, however, it seems to be caused by differences in how they have responded to the specter of FALS. As one estranged cousin explained it, "I just don't go back there [to Danville] anymore. It's too painful." Some family members in Vermont and in Georgia have declined to talk to me about this book.

In his essay "Lay and Professional Knowledge of Genetics and Inheritance," Martin Richards examines the patterns and reasons among the general population for the sporadic and limited knowledge about genetic medicine. As with "medical encounters" in general, he writes, genetic counseling may be very stressful. Ideas—accurate or false, full or limited—may be adopted "as a psychological defense mechanism so the individual can believe that the worst will not happen to them or their children."

Richards discusses common misperceptions about Mendelian genetics, including those theories based on immediate and recent family patterns with which family members are familiar, such as the idea that a disease may skip a generation, or be passed on only from mother to daughter, or seems to strike only first-born daughters, or that it is, as we say, "in the blood."

We tend to mix up our notions of Mendelian genetic inheritance with our general ideas about inheritance and kinship. Family members, therefore, may expect a mix of inherited traits from both father and mother. We say we take after our dad in one respect and our mom in another. We may imagine that a strain may be diluted, and even die out, or that we may get a mild form of it, or a "proneness" that requires a trigger for the disease to manifest itself. There is also, Richards explains, another tendency: "Those who resemble each other physically are seen to be likely to also share a proneness for the disorder which runs in the family." All not true.

Richards calls for a kind of education that is blended into general social education and upbringing, not left to the "top-down" teaching of schools. Families need to understand that autosomal dominant inheritance of disease is like autosomal dominant inheritance of eye color, a single gene characteristic, as differentiated from blended inherited characteristics such as height, or facial appearance. It truly is like a flip of the coin, and the coin flip starts with sexual intercourse.

. . . . .

A number of family members were interviewed for this book. They are of Mary Prior's generation and Curtis Vance's generation, Tennie Toussaint's grandchildren and great-grandchildren. They shared their knowledge, feelings, decisions, relationships, attitudes, and inner lives with me, as those things are affected by the fact that there is a family gene defect and that that defect may someday lead to illness.

Craig Vance is Linda's son and Curtis's brother. When interviewed he was forty-six years old, and a father of two. He and his wife Samantha met in 1998, just before Curtis got sick, and they went through Curtis's year of illness together. Craig's marriage to Sam was his second. He had no children by his first wife and at first he and Sam agreed not to have children, but then they changed their minds. When I interviewed Craig in 2013, his two boys, Normand and Thomas, were ages six and eight.

Craig and Sam had wanted to have kids, he said, but the specter of ALS had held them off. As the effect of Curtis's young death receded in their daily awareness, however, and as Sam's biological clock ticked away, they arrived at a new attitude. "I just decided to live each day as if it were my last," Craig said. "I didn't want to have any regrets about things I had always wanted to do." Having kids is something he had always wanted to do, as well as having fun, working hard and being successful in the family business, and serving his community. As a result, Craig is a very busy man, living a full life.

"Fortunately, I've been successful in business," Craig said, "so if I want to own a Harley, I buy one. If I want a new four-wheeler, I buy one." Craig is president of the family business first started by his grandfather Lane. Over the years, the business has evolved but essentially today it is an excavation business specializing in fiber optic construction, utility pole line construction and other kinds of aerial and underground construction for the communications industry, rock drilling, general excavation, hauling, and trucking. Charles Curtis LLC (named after his two lost brothers) employs nine people. The company also in recent years has responded to the need for storm relief. The company sent trucks and men to New Jersey after Hurricane Sandy in 2012, and has responded to a number of natural disasters since then, usually as a subcontractor replacing utility poles for a larger utility company.

In his community, Craig is a member of the board of selectmen. He is also Worshipful Master of the Masons, head of the local four-wheeler club, and Vice President of VASA, the Vermont All Terrain Sportsman's Association. He is active in little league, to which his company donated a ballfield in North Danville, and other community organizations. He is also a very popular auctioneer, usually donating his time for charity auctions. He has a great sense of humor and a quick wit as an auctioneer, throwing out gags—some on the spot, some well-used—as the items come on the block. Recently he has been raising registered beagles and participating with his sons in field trials.

Craig's children were born after the death of his brother and are still too young to tell about ALS and genes and the family history, but Craig and Sam plan to do that when the time comes.

When Craig was first interviewed, it had been fourteen years since his brother's death. In that time, he had lost his Aunt Mary and cousin Dennis, as reminders of the mutant gene that runs in the family. His plan, however, is to live a full life doing what he likes and what he believes is important.

Craig's cousins Kim and Karen, daughters of Mary and Hollis Prior, lost their mother in 2010 when they were forty-two and thirty-nine respectively. When interviewed in 2013, Kim was forty-five and single, Karen forty-two and the mother of two children ages twelve and nine. Kim lives in Danville, Karen in southwestern Vermont. They both first came face-to-face with the family history of ALS when a member of their own generation, their cousin Curtis, died in 1999.

It is hard to calculate the exact impact of being an FALS family, they said, but the fact is always there. Karen and her husband Roger met in 1995, so they were together when Curtis was sick. They never hesitated to have children, reasoning as many in the family do, that "anything could happen." They are aware not only of the early symptoms of ALS, what to watch for, but also of the specific symptoms of people in the family who have had the disease: their mother's early problem walking, Curtis's legs, and their grandmother Clara's choking. Phantom symptoms, such as general fatigue or even a sore back, lead to the question: Is this it?

Ironically, and in contrast to other diseases in which early detection is crucial, there is no cure or real treatment for ALS, so there is hardly any reason to go to the doctor with a possible symptom of the disease. In fact, they explained, there may be more reasons not to: A) the symptom may go away; B) the symptom may eventually reveal itself to be something else; C) revealing the symptom will alarm your family, probably unnecessarily; D) you may already have self-diagnosed it as something else; E) you may know that ALS is a progressive disease, that that is a key to its diagnosis, so you may just decide to wait and see if, say, another area of muscle weakness develops; and F) there is no cure anyway.

In addition to the patterns of health concerns in the family, there are the other traits of personality, values and tradition. The way they were raised by their parents and the extended family may or may not be products of the family health history. As Kim put it, "We are not a very emotionally expressive family." Certain family members maintain a poker face, even when they are being quite funny or when they are recounting sad events. They don't hug much, the sisters explained, or as Kim put it, "only to irritate others in the family." Is this a result, perhaps evolving over the generations, of all the loss, all that they have had to deal with; or is it a separate inherited personality trait; or is it cultural, a common trait—certainly a feature of the stereotype—among rural people from northern New England? Who knows?

Kim and Karen were raised to be self-sufficient. It was often mentioned that their mother grew up without her mother. "Nobody is going to do it for you," was a common household refrain. Mary was less nurturing and mothering, it seemed, than other mothers. They say that their mother also often said that she was raised by the village of North Danville, and that she was always grateful for the extended family of neighbors and relatives in that hamlet. Perhaps as a result, Mary and Hollis were always very active in their community and church, a value preached by them to their daughters and son Greg. The sisters say that they have reacted against that at times, withdrawing from the community, but Kim has moved back to Danville and is now getting involved there.

Neither of the two sisters has taken definite steps in planning their lives based on their awareness of FALS and their sense of the future. They have not been tested for the SOD1 gene. Their decisions to marry or not, to have children or not, to live their lives cautiously or not, or to make financial plans for their future, have not obviously been affected by the family medical history.

Neither is involved in ALS research, ALS activism, or the family charity—the Curtis Vance Memorial Orchard—except on occasion when asked by their aunts. Their knowledge of ALS and the latest hopes for a cure is sporadic. Ironically, Karen told me, she may know more ALS patients outside of the family than within. Her husband Roger is the manager of a Vermont resort, and through that involvement, they know a number of men who have worked in landscaping and turf care who have contracted ALS and are convinced that it is the exposure to pesticides and herbicides that triggers or causes the disease. The incidence is so high, in fact, that several healthy young men they know are leaving that career to protect their health.

Heather Lynaugh is Susan and Dwayne's daughter, Linda Vance's niece. She was a high school senior when she lost her cousin Curtis in 1999. She is single, lives alone, and works for a division of Merck Pharmaceuticals in Lebanon, New Hampshire. When interviewed in 2013 she said that ALS and the family history do not come together to form a dark cloud over her life, and that ALS has not had a large impact on the decisions she has made in her life, or her life situation today. She has read a little about the disease but she is not a student of it. She notices headlines about ALS, but does not keep a file of clippings.

During her last year of high school, the illness and loss of her beloved cousin was a terribly sad event. She remembers playing basketball with tears in her eyes, everyone wearing green ribbons, and Danville homes with green lights shining in remembrance. She remembers the family's cruise after Curtis's diagnosis, and especially how sad her father was. She became aware at that time of the pattern and the science, and she read a few articles, but she does not follow the latest news of trials or advances. She helps out at the orchard celebration every year, but she is not an activist.

At times, the dark thoughts do intrude. She did read of the high incidence of ALS around Lake Mascoma in Enfield, New Hampshire and became aware that Lebanon's drinking water came from that lake, so for a time she avoided drinking the tap water at her Lebanon apartment, buying bottled water. But after a while, she got tired of that chore and now drinks the water. And there was the morning she woke up after having slept heavily on one arm. The arm felt sore and weak, and she wondered, Is this it? But the symptoms went away during the day. She is usually able to keep the dark thoughts away. In fact, when they do come to her, she might find herself worrying about losing someone else in the family to the disease, not herself, and feeling the sadness that would result from the loss of a beloved cousin again, as well as the sadness of other family members in their grief.

Chuck Longchamp's path to an understanding of the disease and of the odds facing him, is unique. Chuck is Rena Longchamp's grandson, but he was raised by her as a son. As a child he remembers family gatherings at Grammy Tennie's house. He remembers her Glenwood stove, donuts and cookies, the low ceilings of her modest home, and spending time with his cousins in North Danville. Later, his cousins sometimes showed up to listen to his band. Chuck was the drummer, front man, and lead singer for a popular country western band, The Green Mountain Band. He was very busy during the band years, beginning around 1974, with a full-time job and band gigs at night. This was during the period from 1966 through the death of Curtis Vance in 1999 that the family was able to blot out the memories of Clara and Williamina.

When Rena got sick in 1988, Chuck was thirty-five and only somewhat aware of the family disease. He was a married man, but had no children. When he and Susan were dating and contemplating marriage, he told her of the family disease, but the facts were vague and, he said, were not a factor at all as they discussed a life together. There was a disease of some sort that ran in the family, he knew, but whatever it was people thought that it tended to skip a generation, and if that is what caused his mother's death (not a certainty) then maybe it would skip his generation. He was aware that his aunts Clara and Williamina died of the disease in the 1960s, but he was not aware that also in 1988 his mother's sister's son died of the disease in Georgia. When Rena died, he learned about the disease first hand. She knew it was the family disease, he has said.

A few years later, some time in his forties, he recalls, one of his brothers let it slip that actually Chuck was the son of Betty who he thought was his sister. He later learned that other members of the family knew of his actual parentage, but no one told him. Finally, a brother told his wife and she told Chuck. He thinks that his mother Betty, after the death of her mom in 1988, did become a student of the disease. He remembers a folder of research and records, but he hasn't been one to calculate the odds, or to realize the implications of the fact that the woman he thought was his mother, who died of a muscle wasting disease, was actually his grandmother, and the woman he had thought was his sister, who died in her seventies not of a motor neuron disease, was actually his mother. He has never known anything at all about his father, and as far as he knows there were no other offspring from that couple. With the revelation about his actual parentage, Chuck's own chances of inheriting the SOD1 gene defect went from fifty to twenty-five percent, but he hadn't calculated that until interviewed in 2013.

So he was one of the family members who was able to put ALS out of his mind until Curtis got sick. He did not visit Curtis or join in the care circles, but he followed Curtis's case closely. Chuck has kept in touch with the North Danville cousins, has usually attended the orchard celebration and his band has played at it. Chuck is a pleasant, likeable guy who seems to know everyone. He drives an Indian motorcycle, but he no longer plays in the band. Chuck is married, but he and his wife have no children. The reason is not the family history and threat of ALS. Chuck explained that he and his wife Susan were married with an understanding that they would not have children, but that it was due to his busy life, including his music, not the fear of ALS. As he explained it, he really enjoyed his music and his motorcycle, and he had noticed that when men became fathers, they had to abandon pursuits such as those.

As to the impact of being a member of an FALS family, Chuck put himself in the category of his cousins who are aware, not in denial, but not active and not dwelling on it. It is just there. ALS is not a barrier between him and his cousins, but neither is it the glue that binds them.

· · · · ·

In her classic essay "Illness as Metaphor," first published in 1978, Susan Sontag analyzed the metaphorical uses of illness while arguing against the mental habit of finding metaphors to help us understand a disease. Focusing on tuberculosis and cancer, Sontag compared the popular and metaphorical (and contrasting) ways in which we regarded each disease. TB was called "consumption." It was a disease of passion and indulgence, of "too much passion," and it was a disease of the lungs which could perhaps be cured by a change of scenery and air. Cancer is a disease of "lethal growth," usually hidden inside the body, of a spreading infection not associated with any particular organ, likely to start anywhere and spread. In contrast to TB, cancer has been thought of as a disease resulting from the repression of passions. Cancer, at the time that Sontag first wrote, was inexorable, not likely to be cured by a change of scenery. It was always "terminal."

Sontag argues for a "truthful," non-metaphorical way of regarding illness, but metaphor is hard to avoid, as is the process of comparing and contrasting illnesses. We reach for comparisons to describe something that is beyond our experience by comparing it to something that is within our experience. Patients with the disease, such as writers about ALS, courageously attempt to tell us what it is like, for we cannot really know.

"After a year of ALS," wrote Henry Wallace, "you begin to feel like a disembodied spirit in purgatory." With those phrases, Wallace latched on to two of the commonly-felt characteristics of ALS: the loss of the body, and innocence. Wallace feels he is in a hell that he doesn't deserve. Other patients, such as Jenifer Estess, try a prison metaphor: "being in jail . . . for a crime I haven't committed." Perhaps the archetypal character whose profile comes closest to that of the ALS victim is the Biblical Job, the wealthy, successful and blameless man caught in the wager between God and the devil. Job's questioning of his fate and blame forms the core of his meaning.

There is also the pervasive feeling among patients, and their families, that as Wallace put it, "ALS gives you a ringside seat at your own dissolution," as you can fully experience the loss of the strong shell that has held you up and allowed you to move and participate in life. Having that vantage point has resulted in varying attitudes among patients toward the disease and the end of life. Some patients, even if they are not philosophers, become philosophical. Patients of faith may leave their fate in God's hands; others acquire or deepen their faith during their final year. A few choose to take their own lives not long after their diagnosis and before they become severely debilitated. Others choose not to go on life-sustaining machines. Others do not accept this "fate," choosing to fight till the end.

For the Farrs, there is a legacy, vague to some, terribly clear and real to others. The sickness will strike again; they can only look around at family gatherings and wonder whom it will strike. Several family members who have been interviewed for this book actually hope it will be themselves rather than someone else. In the meantime, they try to stay in touch with the experts, with the best in the field, in hopes that a treatment or even a cure is to be found in one of the many clinical trials now just beginning, or in a compound being administered to a symptomatic mouse, or being studied under a powerful microscope. Perhaps a brilliant scientist somewhere has an idea that is the right one. They can hope as a prominent SOD1 family that SOD1 remains a central focus in the search. It sometimes seems, through the ups and downs of trials and news bulletins, as if hope is the only drug that works for them. In the meantime, the learning will continue, as will the fundraising for a cure, the education of family and others, the efforts to memorialize those lost, and the legacy of support for the stricken.

List of Sources by Chapter

Introduction

William Osler, M.D. "Heredity in Progressive Muscular Atrophy as Illustrated in the Farr Family of Vermont." *Archives of Medicine* 4 (1880): 316-320.

Genealogy: Susan Lynaugh, Linda Vance and Mary Prior.

Valerie Cwik. "What is Amyotrophic Lateral Sclerosis," in *Amyotrophic Lateral Sclerosis: A Guide for Patients and Families*, Hiroshi Mitsumoto, MD, ed. (New York: Demos Medical Publishing, 2009).

What is ALS?

Valerie Cwik. "What is Amyotrophic Lateral Sclerosis" in *Amyotrophic Lateral Sclerosis: A Guide for Patients and Families*.

Chapter 1 – Erastus I

A. R. G. Owen. *Hysteria, Hypnosis and Healing: The Work of J.-M. Charcot* (New York: Garrett Publications, 1971).

Georges Guillain. *J.-M. Charcot 1825-1893: His Life – His Work* (New York: Paul B. Hoebner, 1959).

Stanley Finger. *Minds Behind the Brain: A History of the Pioneers and Their Discoveries,* (New York: Oxford University Press, 2000).

Harvey Cushing. *The Life of Sir William Osler, 1869-1939,* (London: Oxford University Press, 1940).

Charles G. Roland. The Dictionary of Canadian Biography Online, accessed at www.biographi.ca/009004-119.01-e.php?id_nbr=7631

Madelaine Brown. "The Wetherbee Ail: The Inheritance of Progressive Muscular Atrophy as a Dominant Trait in Two New England Families," *New England Journal of Medicine* 245 No. 17. October 25, 1951.

"Descendents of John," a family genealogy compiled by Mary Prior and others.

Early Symptoms

Hiroshi Mitsumoto. *Amyotrophic Lateral Sclerosis: A Guide for Patients and Families,* (New York: Demos Health, 2009).

Linda Vance, interview, May 23, 2011.

Jonathan Eig. *Luckiest Man: The Life and Death of Lou Gehrig* (New York: Simon and Schuster, 2005).

Jenifer Estess and Valerie Estess. *Tales from the Bed* (New York: Washington Square Press, 2004).

Chapter 2 – Wesley Ora

Stanley Finger. *Minds Behind the Brain: A History of the Pioneers and Their Discoveries.*

William G. Spiller. "Diseases of the Motor Tracts," in *Modern Medicine: Its Theory and Practice*, ed. William Osler, (Philadelphia: Lea and Febriger, 1910).

Suzanne White Junot. "FDA and Clinical Drug Trials: A Short History," originally published in *A Quick Guide to Clinical Trials,* Madhu Davis and Faiz Kerimani, ed. (Washington: Bioplan, Inc., 2008). 22-55. Accessed 5/23/13 at www.fda.gov/AboutFDA/WhatWeDo/History/Overviews/ucm304485.htm.

Nahum Glatzer. *Franz Rosenzweig: His Life and Thought* (New York: Schocken Books, 1953).

Stanford Encyclopedia of Philosophy. (accessed 5/25/13) http://plato.stanford.edu/entries/rosenzweig.

The Diagnosis

Valerie Cwik. "What is Amyotrophic Lateral Sclerosis," in *A Guide for Patients.*

Donald W. Mulder. "Amyotrophic Lateral Sclerosis: Pitfalls of the Diagnostic Interview," in *ALS – From Charcot to The Present and Into the Future*, F. Clifford Rose ed. (London: Smith-Gordon, 1994).

Hiroshi Mitsumoto. "The Clinical Features and Prognosis of Amyotrophic Lateral Sclerosis," in *A Guide for Patients and Families.*

Chapter 3 – Wesley's Children

Jonathan Eig. *Luckiest Man: The Life and Death of Lou Gehrig.*

Suzanne White Junot. "FDA and Chemical Drug Trials: A Short History."

Barron H. Lerner. *When Illness Goes Public: Celebrity Patients and How We Look at Medicine*. (Baltimore: Johns Hopkins University Press, 2006).

Lawrence Lavine et. al. "Amyotrophic Lateral Sclerosis/Parkinsonism-Dementia Complex in Southern Guam: Is It Disappearing?" *Advances in Neurology*, 56 (1991).

Kathleen McAuliffe. "Are Toxins in Seafood Causing ALS, Alzheimer's, and Parkinson's?" *Discover Magazine*, (May 2011).

Wendee Holdcamp. "Was Lou Gehrig's ALS Caused by Tap Water?" *The Pacific Standard*, January 5, 2012.

Alissa Poh. "Dartmouth Neurology Researchers Probe Murky Waters for Clarity about ALS*," Dartmouth Medicine*, Winter 2011.

Israel S. Wechsler, M.D. "Amyotrophic Lateral Sclerosis," in *A Textbook of Clinical Neurology* (Philadelphia: W.B. Saunders Company, 1958).

Sandra Michelle Farr, email, October 7, 2014.

Bonnie Lavenberg, telephone interview, January 23, 2015.

Obituary, Loriann DeLude, *The Caledonian Record*, May 5, 2009.

The Early Stages

Valerie Cwik, in Mitsumoto ed., *A Guide for Patients.*

Donald W. Mulder, M.D. "Pitfalls of the Diagnostic Interview."

Chapter 4 – Tennie and Her Children

Charlie Myrick, interviews, November 1, 2011, June 6, 2012.

Records, Town of St. Johnsbury, VT.

Tennie Toussaint. "Danville," *Vermont History*, July 1955.

Peggy Pearl, interview

Catherine Beattie, interview, March 26-27, 2014

Tim Ide, interviews

Mary Ide Swainbank, interviews

Arlene Hubbard, interview, April 13, 2013.

Linda Vance, interview, May 23, 2012

Diane McKenna-Yasek, interview, August 28, 2012.

Henry A. Wallace. "Reflection of an ALSer." Unpublished manuscript provided by the Wallace family.

"Pioneer Hi-Bred, " website at www.pioneer.com/home/site/about/business/who-we-are/our-heritage.

John C. Culver and John Hyde, *American Dreamer: A Life of Henry A. Wallace* (New York: W.W. Norton & Co. 2000).

Schlesinger, Arthur. "Who Was Henry A. Wallace," *Los Angeles Times*, March 12, 2000.

The Disease Progresses

Yvonne K. Fulbright. "ALS & Your Sex Life," accessed at Disaboom; http://www.disaboom.com/sexuality-and-disability/als-your-sex-life

Kate E. Dalton. "Nutrition Intervention," in Mitsumoto, ed, *A Guide for Patients*.

Massachusetts General Hospital ALS Multidisciplinary Clinic. Accessed at http://www.massgeneral.org/als/patienteducation/ALS_ sexualityintimacy.aspx

Chapter 5 – Kelly and Rena

Brenda Peterson, interview, April 27, 2013.

Scott Latham, interviews, April 25, 2013, November 11, 2013.

Cindy Hamilton, interview, April 30, 2013.

Chuck Longchamps, interviews, September 19, 2013, July 2, 2013.

Records, Town of St. Johnsbury, accessed June 18, 2013.

Dr. John Ajamie, phone interview, August 25, 2-14

Robert H. Brown Jr. Proceedings of the International Alliance of the ALS/MND Association. Ask the Experts Panel Discussion. November 2001, Oakland, CA.

H.P. "Obituary of Dr. Madelaine Brown," *The New England Journal of Medicine*, October 10, 1968. Courtesy of Massachusetts General Hospital.

Madelaine R. Brown. "Wetherbee Ail: The Inheritance of Progressive Muscular Atrophy in Two New England Families," *The New England Journal of Medicine*, Vol. 245, No. 17, October 25, 1951.

Israel Wechsler, *A Textbook of Clinical Neurology*, 4th Ed Revised. (New York: W.B. Saunders Co, 1939, and the 8th Edition, 1958.)

Elizabeth Cooney, "The Path to a Cure: ALS Specialist Dr. Robert H. Brown Joins Elite Team at UMass." The *Worcester Telegram and Gazette*, December 1, 2008. Accessed at www.thefreelibrary.com.

"H. Robert Horoviz" an autobiographical piece written and published on the Nobelprize.org web site at http://www.nobelprize.org/nobel_prizes/medicine/laureates/2002/horvitz-autobio.html

Robert H. Brown. Transcript of a talk given at Amherst College, June 2008. Accessed at: https://www.amherst.edu/aboutamherst/ news/specialevents/commencement/speeches_multimedia/2008/ honorands/brown/node/53653

Robert H. Brown Jr, et.al. "Gene Linkage in Familial Amyotrophic Lateral Sclerosis: A Progress Report," *Advances in Neurology, Vol. 56 of Amyotrophic*

Lateral Sclerosis and Other Motor Neuron Diseases, edited by Lewis Rowland. Raven Press, 1991.

Robert H. Brown et al., "Linkage of a Gene Causing Familial Amyotrophic Lateral Sclerosis to Chromosome 21 and Evidence of Genetic-Locus Heterogeneity," *The New England Journal of Medicine*. 324: 1381-1384. May 16, 1991.

Robert H. Brown et al., "Mutations in Cu/Zn superoxide dismutase gene are associated with familial amyotrophic lateral sclerosis," *Nature* Vol. 362. March 4, 1993.

Robert G. Miller, Deborah Gelinas, Patricia O'Connor. *Amyotrophic Lateral Sclerosis*. (New York: American Academy of Neurology Press. Demos Publishing. 2005).

Hiroshi Mitsumoto, ed. *Amyotrophic Lateral Sclerosis: A Guide for Patients and Families*.

Robert H. Brown Jr. Proceedings of the International Alliance of the ALS/MND Association. Ask the Experts Panel Discussion. November 2001, Oakland, CA.

Lisa Kinsley, "Genetic Testing for ALS," Neuromuscular Disorders Program of Northwestern University, accessed at http://alsa.org/about-als/genetic-testing-for-als.html

Palliative Care

Hiroshi Mitsumoto, *A Guide for Patients*.

High-tech home, the Steve Saling Residence at the Leonard Florence Center, accessed at http://www.leonardflorencecenter.org

Kay Lazar, "Fighting ALS, One Patient at a Time," *The Boston Globe*, August 14, 2010.

BrainGate website, accessed at http://braingate2.org/braingateSystem.asp

Chapter 6 – Curtis

Linda Vance, interview, February 2, 2012, February 20, 2012

Craig Vance, interview, May 8, 2013

Heidi McCann. Keynote Speech to the Say it With Flowers Benefit, October 1, 2009. Online at: http://www.loomischaffee.org/uploaded/Alumni_photos/Heidi_ALS_speech.pdf

Heidi Vance. *The North Star Monthly*, May 1999.

Anne Wallace Allin. "Family Turns to Healing Circles in Battle Against Lou Gehrig's Disease," *The Caledonian Record*, May 27, 1999.

G. Bensimon et.al. "A Controlled Trial of Riluzole in Amyotrophic Lateral Scleorosis," *The New England Journal of Medicine*, March 3, 1994.

Hiroshi Mitsumoto, Ed. *Amyotrophic Lateral Sclerosis: A Guide for Patients and Families*.

Robert G. Miller et al., *Amyotrophic Lateral Sclerosis*.

Hollis Prior, interview, February 7, 2013.

Merit Cudkowicz, M.D., interview, January 27, 2011.

John Borchardt. "Amgen Neuroscience Research Targets Nervous System Disorders," *The Scientist*, November 6, 2000. Accessed at www.the-scientist.com/?articles.view/articleNo/20116/title/Amgen-neuroscience-research-targets-nervous-system-disorders.

Barry Stavro. "Amgen, Regeneron Say BDNF Isn't Effective," *Los Angeles Times*, January 11, 1997. Accessed at: http://articles.latimes.com/1997-01-11/business/fi-17471_1_side-effects.

Website for MASHNorth, the Metaphysical and Spiritual Healing organization, accesses at http://www.mashnorth.org/als/index.html

National Institute of Health, at www.ncbi.nlm.nih.gov/pubmed/8143712.

John Coffin, interview, January 9, 2014.

Emily Stone. "A Celebration of Life – and Love: Danville Woman Throws Reception for Husband Claimed by ALS," *The Burlington Free Press*, May 20, 2000.

Linda Vance. "A Letter to Curtis Roger Vance ~ Son, Brother, Husband, Relative and Friend," *The North Star Monthly*, January, 2000.

Obituary, Curtis Roger Vance, *The Caledonian Record*, December 21, 1999.

Susan Lynaugh, interview, March 5, 2013.

Curtis Vance Memorial Orchard website accessed at http://www.memorialorchard.com.

Crisis and the End of Life Decision

Barbara Ellen Thompson, N. Michael Murphy, and Mary Eleanor Toms. "Hospice Care," in Mitsumoto, ed, *A Guide for Patients*.

Japan and ALS, accessed at http://www.bioethics.jp/licht_advals.html

Mark R. Glasberg. "Amyotrophic Lateral Sclerosis: Legal and Ethical Issues," in Clifford Rose, ed, *ALS – From Charcot to the Present*.

Chapter 7 – Mary and Dennis

Hollis Prior, interviews, January 7, January 21, 2013.

Kim Darling, "Citizens of the Year Share Work, Fun," *The Caledonian Record*, July 28, 1999.

Bernier Mayo, interview, February 12, 2013.

Dave Redmond, interview, February 26, 2013.

Shay Totten. "Going Once, Twice: Vermont Milk Company Auctions off Assets," *Seven Days*, August 6, 2008. Accessed at www.7dvt.com/2010going-once-twice-vt-milk-company-auctions-assets.

Jeanne Miles. "Businessman Fights ALS with Courage, Humor," *The Caledonian Record*, December 1,2009.

Dr. Sharon Fine, Progress Notes, April 21, 2009 thru December 13, 2011.

Mary Prior, interviews, January 20, April 7, May 6, 2010.

Sharon Fine, interview, October 9, 2013

Linda Vance, interview, February 20, 2012.

Dennis Myrick, interview, January 10, 2010.

CytRx 2008 Annual Report. Accessed at www.cytrx.com

Linda Greensmith, et.al. *Journal of Neurochemistry* Volume 107, Issue 2, (October 2008).

ISIS Pharmaceuticals. Acccessed at www.isispharm.com/Antisense-Technology/index.htm

Margaret Wahl."ISIS-SOD1-Rx: So Far, So Good*," MDA/ALS Newsmagazine*. April 27, 2011.

Amy Labbe. "ALS SOD1Trial: A Watershed Moment," *Quest Magazine: MDA's Research and Health Magazine* March 5, 2010.

Compassionate Care. Accessed at http://www.ccals.org/history.php

Mitsumoto, Hiroshi Ed. *Amyotrophic Lateral Sclerosis: A Guide for Patients and Families.*

Dr. Merit Cudkowicz, interview, Massachusetts General Hospital, January 27, 2011.

Dr. Tim Tanner, interview, January 11, 2013.

Ro Myrick, interviews, August 8, February 11, 2013.

BrainGate company website, acccessed at braingate2.org.

Clinical Trials

National Institutes of Health, Glossary definition. Accessed at https://clinicaltrials.gov/ct/help/glossary /phase

Amy Elllis Nutt and Brady Dennis. "ALS Patients Press FDA for Quick Access to Controversial Biotech Drug," *The Washington Post*, April 3, 2015.

Chapter 8 – Clif and the Ice Bucket Challenge

Lee Beattie, interview, August 29, 2014.

Clif Langmaid, interviews, September 7, October 29, 2013, May 10, June 19, 2014.

Peter Schworn. "Effort Aims to Put ALS on Ice," *The Boston Globe,* August 13, 2014.

Denise Lavoie. "Soaked for Charity: Ice Bucket Challenges Get Cool," *The Caledonia Record*, August 14, 2014 (AP story).

Taylor Reed. "Community, Family Fight Deadly Disease," *The Caledonian Record*, September 17, 2014.

Taylor Reed. "Family Plays Role in ALS Research Breakthrough," *The Caledonian Record*, September 17, 2014.

Susan Lynaugh. "Family Speaks of ALS Battles," *The Caledonian Record*, September 17, 2014.

Paul Hayes. "Community Rallies to ALS Challenge, Local Family," *The Caledonian Record*, September 22, 2014.

Kitty Toll, interview, June 19, 2015.

Susan Lynaugh, interviews, November 20, 2013, February 19, 2014.

Linda Vance, interview, November 21, 2013.

"Immunosuppression in Amyotrophic Lateral Sclerosis." Accessed at Clinical Trials.gov.

Tom Henderson. "Ted Harada: His ALS Miracle Continues to Amaze." Accessed at crainsdetroit.com.

Miriam Falco,"Patient, Doctors Encouraged by ALS Trial," CNN, September 28, 2011.

Obituary, "Clifton F. 'Clif' Langmaid," *The Caledonian Record*, August 9, 2014.

Alexandra Sifferlin. "Here's How the ALS Ice Bucket Challenge Actually Started," *Time,* August 18, 2014.

CBS News. "Putting 'Ice Bucket Challenge' Cash Into Action," November 18, 2014, 7:00 AM. Accessed at www.massgeneral.org/als/default.aspx

Marketwatch. "Five Companies that Will Get a Boost from Ice Bucket Challenge," *The New York Post*, August 22, 2014.

"The ALS Association Announces Initial Commitment of $21.7 Million from Ice Bucket Challenge Donations to Expedite Search for Treatments and a Cure for ALS." Press release accessed at www.alsa.org/news/media/press-releases/ibc-initial-commitment.html

The Promise of Genetics – Going to Be Tested

Lisa Kinsley. "Genetic Testing for ALS," Neuromuscular Disorders Program of Northwestern University. Accessed at http://alsa.org/about-als/genetic-testing-for-als.html

Lisa Kinsley, telephone interview, November 26, 2013.

Chapter 9 – Hope and Defeat, Advances and Setbacks

Author's notes, ALS TDI Leadership Summit, November 1, 2012, The Sheraton Boston Hotel, Boston, MA.

The Orphan Disease Act. Accessed at http://history.nih.gov/research/downloads/PL107-280.pdf

Prevalence of ALS, Hiroshi Mitsumoto, *A Guide for Patients*.

Famous People Who Died of ALS. Accessed at www.alsmndalliance.org/famous_people.html

Douglas Martin. "Jenifer Estess, 40; Fought Lou Gehrig's Disease," *New York Times*, December 17, 2003.

Clinical Trials. Accessed at clinicaltrials.gov

David Hochman. "Feelin' Alright, Oh, Yeah,*" AARP, The Magazine*, April/May 2013.

The Orphan Disease Act. Accessed at http://www.fda.gov/RegulatoryInformation/Legislation/FederalFoodDrugandCosmeticActFDCAct/SignificantAmendmentstotheFDCAct/OrphanDrugAct/default.htm

Biogen Idea and Dexpramipexole. *The Boston Globe* at www.bostonglobe.com/business/2012/04/04/biogen-idec-says-drug-for-lou-gehrig-disease-far-from-long-shot/QNeQsv5vKBTi8eBCJmFouL /story.html

Steve Perrin. Accessed at www.partneringforcures.org/media_center/slides/ALSTherapyDevInst.pda

Augie Nieto and T.W. Pearson. *Augie's Quest: One Man's Journey from Success to Significance*. (New York: Bloomsbury USA. 2007).

Isis Pharmaceuticals and Anti-Sense. Accessed at www.isispharm.com/Pipeline/Current-Advances.htm

Three Sisters, HBO.

Stephen Hawking. Accessed at www.upi.com/Odd_News/2013/01/01/Stephen-Hawking-conjures-black-hole-in-ad/UPI-35841357080414.

Jonathan Weiner. *His Brother's Keeper: One Family's Journey to the Edge of Medicine.* (New York: Harper Collins, 2004).

Obituary, "Michael Zaslow, 54, Soap Actor; Publicized Lou Gehrig's Disease," *The New York Times*, December 9, 1998.

Jenifer Estess. *Tales from the Bed: A Memoir.* (New York: Washington Square Press, 2004).

Biogen Idec Failed Trial. Accessed at www.bloomberg.com/news/2013-01-03/biogen-sinks-as-als-drug-fails-to-show-efficacy-in-trial.html.

Robert Weisman. "Biogen Idec's ALS Drug Falls Short in Trials," *The Boston Globe*. January 3, 2013.

Rob Goldstein, interview February 14, 2013.

Worldwide Estimates. Accessed at www.alscounts.com/livingpatients.html

Alice Park. *The Stem Cell Hope: How Stem Cell Medicine Can Change Our Lives,* (New York: Hudson Street Press, 2011).

Tom Henderson, "Ted Harada: His ALS Miracle Continues to Amaze; Stem-Cell Protesters are Blind to the Big Picture," *Crains Detroit Business*, May 3, 2013. Accessed at www.crainsdetroit.com/ article/20130503/BLOG007/130509948/#

Stem Cell Trial, University of Michigan. Accessed at http://www.uofmhealth.org/news/archive/201304/fda-approves-phase-ii-stem-cell-trial-als-led-u-ms-dr-eva

Carolyn Y. Johnson. "Gene Therapy's Time Seems to Have Come," *The Boston Globe*, July 14, 2013.

Carl Zimmer, "The Fall and Rise of Gene Therapy," *Wired*, September 2013.

ISIS. Website http://isispharm.com/Antisense-Technology/Antisense-Drug-Discovery-Platform/Basic-Science.htm

Amy Labbe, *MDA Magazine*, March 5, 2010. Accessed at http://quest.mda.org/news/als-sod1-trial-%E2%80%98watershed-moment%E2%80%99

Dr. Merit Cudkowicz, telephone interview, April 4, 2013.

Timothy Miller, M.D. e.al, "An antisense oligonucleotide against *SOD1* delivered intrathecally for patients with *SOD1* familial amyotrophic lateral sclerosis: a phase 1, randomised, first-in-man study," *The Lancet Neurology*, Early Online Publication, 29 March 2013.

Dr. Frank Bennett, ISIS Pharmaceuticals, telephone interview, April 16, 2013.

Blocking Immune Cells, website of ALS TDI, www.als.net/ALS-Research/166/ClinicalTrials.

ALS TDI and Gilenya. Accessed at www.als.net/Media/5428/News/

"How Gilenya Works." Accessed at www.gilenya.com/c/how-gilenya-works

Enrique Reynaud. "Protein Misfolding and Degenerative Diseases," *Scitable by Nature Education*, 3(9) 28.

"Amorfix Announces Progress on ALS Program." Accessed at www.amorfix.com/pr_2013-03-20.php, March 20, 2013.

Patrick Freund et al. "Anti-Nogo-A Antibody Treatment Promotes Recovery of Manual Dexterity after Unilateral Cervical Lesion in Adult Primates – Re-examination and Extension of Behavioral Data," *The European Journal of Neuroscience*, March 2009 . 29(5). Accessed at www.ncbi.nlm.nih.gov/pubmed/19291225 on May 31, 2013.

Neurotone. Accessed at www.neurotune.com/tl_files/neurotune/news/PR_ALS-Neurotune_ 20120514.pdf

Mexiletine. Accessed at website of ALS TDI on June 6, 2013 at http://blogs.als.net/post/2013/02/05/ Mexiletine-channeling-ALS.aspx

"Neudexta: Getting More than Emotional" Rob Goldstein, interview, August 26, 2013, and http://blogs.als.net/post/Nuedexta-getting-more-than-emotional.aspx

Wim Robberecht and Thomas Phillips. "The Changing Scene of Amyotrophic Lateral Sclerosis," *Nature Reviews – Neuroscience*, 14, 248-264 (April 2013)> Accessed online March 6, 2013 at www.nature.com/nrn/journal/v14/n4/abs/ nrn3430.html

Lauren LeBano. "NFL PLayers Have High Mortality Rate from Alzheimer's Disease and ALS," *Neurology Reviews*, 2012. Accessed at www.neurologyreviews.com/home/article/nfl-players-have-high-mortality-rate-from-alzheimer-s-disease-and-als/c4ebca691f0efea9efb047ebc8c48d9e.html

Dr. Elijah Stommel, interview, January 23, 2014.

Number of SOD1 mutations. Teepu Siddique et.al. "Age and Founder Effect of SOD1 A4V Mutation Causing ALS," *Neurology* May 12, 2009. 72(19). 1634-1639. Accessed at http://www.ncbi.nlm.nih.gov/pmc/articles/PMC2683645/ July 12, 2013.

Martin R. Turner et al. "Controversies and Priorities in Amyotrophic Lateral Sclerosis," *Lancet Neurology*, 12 (3), March 2013.

C9orf72. ALS Association News, "New Genetic Mutation Identified: the Most Common Cause of FTD and ALS Accounting for as much as One Third of

All Familial ALS, September 21, 2011 at www.alsa.org/news/archive/9p21-abnormality.html

Bradley N. Smith et. al, "The C9orf72 Expansion Mutation is a Common Cause of ALS+/-FTD in Europe and Has a Single Founder," European Journal of Human Genetics (2013) 21. Published online 13 June 2012, and accessed at http://www.nature.com/ejhg/journal.v21/n1/full/ejhg201298a.html

Amorfix Life Sciences. "Amorfix Confirms Presence of Misfolded SOD1 in Sporadic ALS," http://www.amorfix.com/pr_2013-10-24.php

Dr. Robert H. Brown Jr., interview, August 26, 2013.

Voyager Therapeutics. Accessed at http://www.voyagertherapeutics.com/programs.php

White House initiative. Accessed at http://www.whitehouse.gov/the-press-office/2015/01/30/fact-sheet – president-obama-s-precision-medicine-initiative

To Be a FALS Family

Lisa Kinsley, telephone interview, January 29, 2014.

Hiroshi Mitsumoto, ed. *A Guide for Patients.*

Chapter 10 – Bargaining with the Devil

Genetic Medicine and ALS. Accessed at http://www.alsa.org/about-als/genetic-testing-for-als.html

Dr. Robert H. Brown Jr, interview, August 26, 2013.

Diane McKenna-Yasek, PowerPoint. Accessed at http://www.alsmndalliance.org/uploads/Polak.pdf

Martin Richards, "Lay and Professional Knowledge of Genetics and Inheritance," *Public Understanding of Science*, 1996 5:217.

Craig Vance, interviews, May 8, 2013, January 24, 2014.

Kim Prior and Karen Hill, interview, July 5, 2013.

Heather Lynaugh, interview, August 20, 2013.

Chuck Longchamps, interview, September 19, 2013.

Susan Sontag, *Illness as Metaphor*, (New York: McGraw Hill, 1978).

Henry A. Wallace, "Reflections of an ALSer." Used with permission of the Wallace family.

Acknowledgments

I want to express my gratitude and admiration to all of the members of the Farr family who told me their stories. All of those stories were painful to relive. Three members of the family have died of ALS since I began my research and writing; all three welcomed me into their homes and told me with courage and good spirit of their first symptoms, their decisions and feelings, and their hopes for future generations. I especially want to thank Linda Vance and Susan Lynaugh, two sisters who have lost a sister and a brother, their mother, two aunts, three cousins, and their grandmother—all to ALS—during their lifetimes. Hardest of all to imagine is the experience of losing a young son, as Linda did, but she agreed to tell me, through her tears, what it was like. Charlie Myrick was an invaluable source of information and family history—the only member of his generation whom I had the privilege of interviewing. Clif Langmaid's cousin and companion Lee Beattie also shared facts and feelings about her life and work with Clif.

Other Vermont family members who have agreed to be interviewed for this book include Rosaleen Myrick, Robert McGill Jr, Chuck Longchamps, and Bonnie Lavenberg. Hollis Prior told me about his life with Mary. Members of the next generation, Curtis's brothers and cousins Craig Vance, Kim Prior, Karen Hill, Maureen Myrick, and Heather Lynaugh told me of their experiences and how they live their lives under the cloud of ALS. In Georgia, I learned from Scott Latham, Joanna Freeman, Thomas Ralston and Cindy Lou Hamilton, and in Pennsylvania Brenda Peterson and her daughter Wendy Kolb—all descendants of Viola Ralston.

Sandra Michelle Farr from Virginia, a tireless ALS activist and family genealogist, a member of another branch of the Farr family, met with me and continued to provide advice and suggestions for my research.

Two important neurologists in the search for a cure for ALS—and in the care and counseling of Farr family members—took the time to meet with me and guide me. Dr. Robert H. Brown Jr, the scientist who found the family gene, met with me, along with his colleague Diane McKenna-Yasek at the University of Massachusetts Medical Center in Worcester, Massachusetts. Dr. Merit Cudkowicz of Massachusetts General Hospital, who has treated four members of the family, invited me to visit her clinic and to be interviewed on several occasions. Dr. Elijah Stommel of Dartmouth Hitchcock Medical Center in Lebanon, New Hampshire guided me to an understanding of environmental issues. At the ALS Therapy Development Institute in Cambridge, Massachusetts, Rob Goldstein informed me of ALS TDI's programs and therapies, and guided me in highlighting the latest and most promising developments in the search for a cure.

Local physicians John Ajamie, Tim Tanner, and Sharon Fine shared their recollections (and sometimes their notes) of their treatment of Rena, Curtis, Mary, and Dennis. Neurologist Dr. Parker Towle, retired surgeon Dr. Jerry Rankin, and general practitioner Dr. Tom Ziobrowski each read sections of the manuscript. ALS patient Joe Newell, not a Farr family member or FALS patient, welcomed me into his home.

Many members of the Danville community shared with me their memories of the Farr family, North Danville village life, and the history of the town. They include Kate Beattie, Shirley Langmaid, Arlene Hubbard, Tim Ide, and Jenness Ide.

Readers of the whole manuscript who helped me with proofreading, style issues, and in finding a way to write about ALS for the general reader, were Anne Brooks, Terry Hoffer, and my devoted and supportive wife Mary Swainbank.

To those members of the family who did not want to be interviewed for this book: I certainly understand your wish to live your lives without reminders and memories of the family history, and I hope that I have faithfully and sensitively described that history.

About the Author

The Farr Disease is Dan Swainbank's second book. A former high school and college writing teacher, Dan is also the author of *Mr. Vail is in Town: Theodore N. Vail, AT&T and His Lyndon Legacy.* He writes about national and international history with chapters based in northeastern Vermont. Dan lives in North Danville, Vermont.

www.ingramcontent.com/pod-product-compliance
Lightning Source LLC
Chambersburg PA
CBHW071654200326
41519CB00012BA/2511